PERFECTING
SMILES
CHANGING LIVES

PERFECTING SMILES

CHANGING LIVES

YOUR GUIDE TO
AN EXCEPTIONAL DENTAL EXPERIENCE

DR. AMI BARAKAT

Published by Advantage, Charleston, South Carolina.
Member of Advantage Media Group.

ADVANTAGE is a registered trademark, and the Advantage colophon is a trademark of Advantage Media Group, Inc.

Printed in the United States of America.

10 9 8 7 6 5 4 3 2 1

ISBN: 978-1-59932-975-8
LCCN: 2018939807

Cover design by George Stevens.
Layout design by Megan Elger.

This publication is designed to provide accurate and authoritative information in regard to the subject matter covered. It is sold with the understanding that the publisher is not engaged in rendering legal, accounting, or other professional services. If legal advice or other expert assistance is required, the services of a competent professional person should be sought.

Advantage Media Group is proud to be a part of the Tree Neutral® program. Tree Neutral offsets the number of trees consumed in the production and printing of this book by taking proactive steps such as planting trees in direct proportion to the number of trees used to print books. To learn more about Tree Neutral, please visit **www.treeneutral.com**.

Advantage Media Group is a publisher of business, self-improvement, and professional development books and online learning. We help entrepreneurs, business leaders, and professionals share their Stories, Passion, and Knowledge to help others Learn & Grow. Do you have a manuscript or book idea that you would like us to consider for publishing? Please visit **advantagefamily.com** or call **1.866.775.1696**.

To my wife, Anne,
and my children Kristen, Mikayla, Jordan, and Aaliyah
for your support and for giving me the will to strive
for never-ending improvement.

Table of Contents

Part One: A Category of One

INTRODUCTION 3
YOUR SMILE, OUR PASSION

CHAPTER ONE 15
The Patient-Centric Philosophy

CHAPTER TWO 23
What is an Unhealthy Smile Costing You?

CHAPTER THREE 33
Unleashing Human Potential

CHAPTER FOUR 41
Best Team in Town

CHAPTER FIVE 47
Steward of Your Smile

CHAPTER SIX 59
The Power of a Free Day of Dentistry

CHAPTER SEVEN 65
Begin with the End in Mind

Part Two: Your Mouth at Every Age

CHAPTER EIGHT 73
Childhood

CHAPTER NINE 81
Pre-Teens and Teenagers

CHAPTER TEN 89
Ages 20–39

CHAPTER ELEVEN. 103
Ages 40–59

CHAPTER TWELVE 115
Ages 60+

Part One

A Category of One

Introduction

YOUR SMILE, OUR PASSION

I wanted to be a dentist ever since I was a child. I remember when I was two, jumping up and down on my parents' bed at home in Winnipeg. I lost my balance and fell, slamming face-first on the hard floor. My front tooth was horribly damaged, and it got infected and eventually died. My parents took me to the dentist to get it removed, and the dentist was so great at his job that when I walked out of the office, I told my parents I wanted to be a dentist when I grew up.

And you know what? I've never really wanted to do anything else with my life. Just ask my kindergarten and first-grade teachers. Up to twenty years old, I never found anything else I wanted to do with my life—except play professional hockey or soccer, but I wasn't good enough at those sports to see it as a realistic goal. Being a dentist though—that was a realistic goal.

I was always good at science and biology. When I got braces at ten years old, I discovered how dentistry wasn't just drilling and filling holes and replacing missing teeth; dentists could also straighten teeth. I loved that idea. Both of my parents were engineers, and teeth straightening seemed like a cool mix of dentistry and engineering.

As I grew up, I learned that not only was dentistry something I was passionate about, but it was also a good field to be in to support my family and, at the same time, it would allow me to make a difference in people's lives. People asked me many times along the way if I ever considered becoming a medical doctor. I'd tell them I never really did, because I didn't like the idea of being around death and loss. Instead, as a dentist, I could help people smile brighter and better, which was a better path for me.

I earned my dental degree in 1999, but I've never quit learning since then, especially after I opened my own practice, Villanova Dental Studio, in 2004. As good as dental schools are, they just teach students the basics of dentistry knowledge. It's up to us to expand on that knowledge. The vast majority of dentists just take the bare minimum of continuing education credits to keep their license. But for me, that was never enough; the status quo has never been good enough. There is so much technology, so much research and development, so much more information coming out every year, that if I just continued to practice the same way without striving to do better, I would be left behind.

If there's a better way I can serve my patients, I owe it to myself and I owe it to them to treat them with the best knowledge mankind has to offer. That is why, whether it be the best knowledge or best technology to make procedures less painful or make it easier for the patient, I feel it's my responsibility to always provide that to my patients. I always want to do better.

Beyond "Drill and Fill"

While I learn important information that I incorporate into my practice from every education course I take, one of those sessions changed my practice significantly in 2007.

I was in Las Vegas taking a course on physiologic dentistry (at the Las Vegas Institute for Advanced Dental Studies), which deals with the effects that tooth and jaw position have on the entire body. Physiologic dentistry is a way to treat neuromuscular issues dealing with the misalignment of the jaw and temporomandibular joint disorder (TMJ) that causes pain in the jaw and the muscles that control jaw movement including debilitation headaches. I knew about TMD (temporomandibular dysfunction) and neuromuscular issues; that's why I went to the training. But I didn't realize what I was able to do about those issues within the scope of my license.

At the time, I was just a general and cosmetic dentist, giving exams, doing fillings and crowns and root canals—what most dentists do. That was a pretty good job; after all, I was helping people regain their self-confidence and changing their lives for the better. Like most dentists, however, I was undereducated in how to use a holistic approach in treatment, and in treating not only the teeth and gums, but treating pain, airway issues—the whole body. They simply do not teach that properly in dental school.

But this course in Las Vegas opened my eyes to the breadth of treatment I could provide. Once I learned I could treat the underlining dental issues to prevent or eliminate pain and get sufferers back to where they could function—and that I could make corrections most doctors and neurologists could not because the treatment isn't a part of their scope of practice—I got really excited.

These were significant problems I would be able to help with. TMD can cause headaches, ear congestion, ringing in the ears, neck pain, and a host of other problems. There are hundreds of thousands, if not millions, of people walking around North America with headaches and migraines who have been to a doctor. The doctor gives them medication that offers short-term relief and makes them feel fuzzy. They've been to a chiropractor. They've been to a physiotherapist. At best, those offer temporary solutions, and often they offer no solution.

By treating underlining mouth and airway issues, I would be able to help patients alleviate major problems like mouth breathing, which seems like no big deal but really can be, particularly in children. Mouth breathing—which can be caused by a nasal airway issue and results in a lack of oxygen saturation in the brain—is associated with tooth grinding (bruxism), nightmares or night terrors, restless sleep, restless legs syndrome, bedwetting, and problems in school. It can cause snoring, which is something children shouldn't do. As a result of mouth breathing, kids are waking up tired, restless, and cranky. That will interfere with their ability to focus. So many times, problems like chronic tiredness and lack of ability to focus are diagnosed as attention-deficit/hyperactivity disorder (ADHD); the children are then put on prescription drugs to deal with the problem that can leave them in a fog and not feeling like themselves.

But studies show more than half of children diagnosed with ADHD also mouth breathe, and it's not a coincidence. Often when we can get this type of child's nasal obstruction under control and get them breathing through their nose, the "ADHD" goes away. It turns out it was never ADHD to begin with. It was an airway problem. So, we can also get them off those medications and back to who they naturally are personality-wise. Too many orthodontists identify a moderate or severe issue at this age and choose to wait to treat. That makes no sense to me. In what other medical field do we identify a problem and wait three to five years until it's as bad as it can possibly get and then treat it?

I was just a traditional dentist and I heard about this training, and I thought, "There's got to be something like this that I can do to better serve my patients."

Who better to treat an airway issue than dentists and ENTs? Airway issues are in the same locations where we perform our treatments, after all.

I remember calling my wife from the hotel and talking her ear off for thirty minutes about this new treatment path. I remember telling her, "I'm going to be able to change people's lives and get rid of their pain. When I come back, I'm going to learn how to do all of this."

And I did. I got thorough training so I would know how to treat these problems. As a result of hundreds of additional hours of training, my view as a dentist is outside of the box compared to most dentists. Everyone else is in the box constructed at their university or college, and they don't stray from that very much. They are practicing based on science from the '80s and '90s, but it's 2018 and we now know so much more about how things develop in the mouth, and we know so much more about these disorders.

Now, because of my training, if I detect there's an airway issue that is the underlying cause of a patient's symptoms, I'm able to figure out what the issue is and how to solve it. If it's a problem I can't fix—for example, enlarged adenoids or allergies—then we refer to an ENT specialist or an allergist or a medical doctor to address that problem because it will benefit not only facial development, but also have a host of other benefits.

It has become my life's goal to educate patients and those suffering with these problems on how a properly trained neuromuscular or physiologic dentist can solve their problems, and to educate and treat kids I see in my practice in such a way as to prevent them from ever suffering from these problems. From now until I retire, that's my goal.

It's really rewarding and wonderful to be able to do this for my patients, to not only fix their teeth, but really change their lives by eliminating the pain or breathing issues that limit them in their lives. And it's not just fixing problems with teeth or breathing. For instance, some of my patients have had debilitating migraines. To be able to get rid of that for someone is an extremely amazing thing to do. It's considerably better than doing a filling or a root canal, because I'm really improving their quality of life.

However, a few years later, I noticed something troubling about these migraine treatments. A concern that would change my practice again.

Physiological Orthodontics

Treatment for migraines is in two phases. Phase one is to make a temporary appliance to get the patient comfortable. Phase two is to do crowns, veneers, or orthodontics to make the treatment permanent and lifelong; most patients prefer orthodontics to move the teeth to this new, better, more physiologic position. (You'll learn about the phases in this book.)

Too often, I would get my patients headache free—phase one— and then I would refer them to an orthodontist to move the teeth to the proper position. The orthodontist, however, without the proper neuromuscular training, would lose the bite we established and the symptoms would return. It got to the point where I dreaded referring out to orthodontists.

One day I was sitting on a plane on the way home from a vacation, thinking about a patient who needed a referral. I knew who I was going to refer her to, but it bothered me because of the experience from my previous referrals. Then something clicked within me. I turned to my wife and told her, "When we land, I'm going to do it myself. I'm going to learn how to do orthodontics properly so I don't have to send my healthy patients away and not be sure phase two will be done properly."

And with the same determination I had to become a dentist—the same determination I had to learn physiologic dentistry—I did it. I learned about physiologic orthodontics, and now I handle both phases one and two myself.

Since making that decision, I have taken hundreds of hours of advanced training and really focused my practice on physiologic orthodontics, which takes into account facial beauty, TMJ, and airway (including sleep apnea prevention)—not just straight teeth. It allows me to take holistic dental care to a whole new level.

I hear people say, "But you're not an orthodontist."

To which I say, "You're right, I'm not an orthodontist. I see that as my advantage. My initial training is in TMJ health and facial beauty and I feel that makes me better and more qualified to treat you or your child. Straightening teeth is the easy part!" I say that because I'm much more proactive in terms of health, rather than just focusing on cosmetics.

And I feel the results for my patients are better in many ways. For example, when a kid's mouth has lots of crowding, many traditional orthodontists solve the problem by pulling permanent teeth to create room. In my opinion, that is bordering on malpractice in 99 percent of cases. Rather, most of these cases can and should be treated by creating space for all of the teeth that are meant to be there. Sure, pulling teeth will allow for straight teeth, but it will make for a very narrow smile and crowd the tongue, which forces it back in the mouth and increases the risk for obstructive sleep apnea. This can also force the lower jaw back, increasing the risk of TMD which can include jaw clicking, migraines, jaw pain, and more. It also pulls back the midface, leading to a flatter facial profile. As a result, both esthetics and function are compromised.

Or consider the approach for teenagers. Most orthodontics is based on retraction, on straightening teeth and then pulling them back into the arch and making them straight. It does not take into account so many of the factors that caused the problem to begin with and the problems that the orthodontics could cause, such as obstructive sleep apnea, TMJ problems, and neuromuscular problems. The main goal for most orthodontists—and quite honestly, for most patients—is to get the teeth straight.

But if that was really the only variable, then it would be easy. The problem is, there are so many problems improperly done orthodontics can cause. As I said before, we just can't treat kids today like how we treated them in the 1980s—we know so much more now. We have to do better.

Before we even start treatment at my practice, we look at the person's airway. We consider questions such as: Are they breathing properly through their nose? Is there any obstruction to their airway? Do they have poor oral habits that resulted in improper tongue position or improper cheek position? Was there a bad habit like thumb-sucking?

Finding out those issues allows us to address more than just a tooth-crowding issue.

The whole point of physiologic orthodontics is to take into account all these surrounding variables, and to address them. In

North America, there are only a tiny percentage of orthodontists or dentists who have this physiological philosophy—far less than 5 percent. I think eventually that will change, that more and more will start embracing that holistic philosophy. But change is slow to happen.

Focusing on the Whole Face

Physiological orthodontics is not just about relieving pain, addressing breathing issues, and spacing out teeth crowding. It's not just about producing a beautiful smile; we go even further to craft a beautiful face.

The type of orthodontics we do is called "face forward", which means we develop the upper jaw and the midface. That is the area of the nose and cheekbones, and by developing them, we allow the lower jaw to also develop properly. As an example: Imagine a patient's midface didn't develop properly due to improper breathing as a child. The middle of their face is too sunken in. The nostrils are very tiny and their sinuses never developed because there was no air passing through them. That's not a genetic problem; it's an environmental problem (usually caused by subclinical allergies, inflamed turbinates or adenoids).

If we develop the cheek bones and under the nose, we've found that we can create not only more beautiful teeth, but also more beautiful faces. We do this by using specialized appliances and techniques and making sure we address the underlying cause of the problem to begin with so they develop properly.

As a result, a much lower percentage of patients who have been seeing us since childhood have grown up to have obstructive sleep apnea and TMD.

So, in a nutshell, physiologic orthodontics addresses form and function, addresses aesthetics and beauty, and most importantly, the long-term health and comfort of the patient.

I care about the beauty of your smile, and of your face. I care about your quality of life. That's why our motto here at Villanova Dental Studio is: "Perfecting smiles, changing lives." What we do really does go beyond "drilling and filling."

A Different Experience

As you can see, Villanova is a different dental practice. And I think when you come into the practice, you can tell that right away. You'll see that our office reflects our focus on beauty.

We've created a spa-like experience with a relaxing atmosphere. There is no sliding glass window, no front desk you have to approach to sign in. You walk right into a living room, right into a reception area with a fountain waterfall, a nice big flat-screen TV, and then business offices off to the side. We have a greeter who offers cookies, coffee, water, or juice.

I truly believe if you have the best dentists in the world but they have really poor customer service—there's dust on the walls and old magazines on creaky tables, or even a really bad website—you, the guest, will get the impression you're not in the offices of someone you can trust with your treatment. On the other hand, if we take a below average dentist, and if he spends a little money on an amazing website and presenting a picture-perfect, clean practice, people will think, "He must be good because it's really clean and nice in here." Offices speak to you; they're the first impression you'll have of the person who will be in your face for the duration of your procedure, the first impression of this person who will be advising you on the best course of dental action.

So, we are trying to match the quality of care you will receive to the experience you will get when you walk into our offices. Am I as concerned about how my office presents as I am about how you'll look and feel after treatment? No. But it's close. I want my offices to reflect the care that we take with your treatment.

About This Book

I hope that as you read the rest of this book, you realize that not all dental practices are created equal. The level and devotion to training and the effort put into making the dental experience a unique and excellent one varies by dentist. And I truly believe that here at Villanova, we're the best.

I hope you understand that dentistry isn't the way you remember it from your childhood—or shouldn't be, at any rate. So much has changed, and there are so many different ways to make the dental experience great, and so many ways for you to access the best dental care the world has to offer all in one place.

I feel very fortunate. I had a great upbringing and had every opportunity to pursue my passion and my dream. I know not everyone has that opportunity. I really believe in second chances, and especially in giving youths an opportunity, at least part of the opportunity I had, to succeed in their life. That's why we provide scholarships for underprivileged youth to go on to post-secondary education. That's why I participate in Dentistry from the Heart, which is discussed later in this book. Those are just a couple of the charitable ways we give back to the community. We also sponsor several hockey and soccer teams, because even if I can't play professionally, I can still contribute to others who may want to when they grow up.

Part two of the book talks about different dental conditions associated with each age and stage of life. You can flip to it and check out the normal issues and conditions for people your age or your child's age any time you want. It's great because you don't need to call the dentist's office or wonder if something's wrong. It includes a lot of common questions patients ask at every age, and, quite honestly, a lot of questions patients don't ask and just assume the answer to—and unfortunately, they typically assume wrong. I cannot count how many times a parent has said to me, "Maybe I should wait until they're older and all the permanent teeth are in before getting braces." In those cases, I mention that the dental associations recommend the first orthodontic visit by age seven because that is when you can do phase one treatment and really affect their jaw development and their jaw growth for the better. That is in this section too.

I think you'll find the entire book very helpful, informative, and enjoyable to read. And I hope you'll look at dentistry a little differently after reading this book. It's a little piece of me, a way for you to get to know me. Hopefully, I'll get to know you, too.

Enjoy! And remember, at Villanova Dental Studio, we are perfecting smiles and changing lives.

Chapter One

THE PATIENT-CENTRIC PHILOSOPHY

Tell me if this sounds familiar: You open the door to a medical office and the first thing you notice is the harsh smell of disinfectant. There are a bunch of old, worn out chairs lining the walls—none of which are comfortably facing the television screen that's displaying static—and stacks of outdated lifestyle magazines are scattered on the scarce side tables. And at the furthest end of the room is a sliding glass window, scratched and smudged with fingerprints. Behind them sits an assistant who somehow doesn't see you standing at said window for at least two or three minutes after you've arrived.

At some point, we came to accept this kind of treatment as the norm; that we weren't people as much as we were penitents, come to beg for a moment of time with the almighty Doctor, and even if we'd scheduled an appointment, we were willing to wait for hours—half our day, even—for what ultimately amounts to five minutes of attention.

This is not how it should be.

Five Reasons People Don't Like Doctor Visits

From the Huffington Post

1. The doctor doesn't listen

2. The long wait

3. The doctor doesn't care

4. The doctor makes too much money

5. My dog gets more respect

A large part of the dissatisfaction with doctor visits is created by the environment and the doctor's non-patient-centric approach to delivering treatment. Most people's perception of a medical office, in other words, is that sliding glass window, the clipboard of medical questions, and the long wait until you're beckoned behind the door and into a treatment room. From the moment patients step in the front door, they're treated like a piece of paperwork because in the end, that's really all they're seen as.

The Patient-Centric Model

Our office couldn't be further from this dated, frustrating approach. For one, we don't even *have* a sliding glass window.

Words that Describe a Patient-Centric Model

Comfortable

Relaxed

Understood

Important

Satisfied

Listened to

Cared for

Respected

The system we have created in our office is what's called the Patient-Centric Model. The entire experience is crafted around putting the patient first, with predetermined steps that include speed when speed is necessary, clear communication, and treatment that is well above the norm.

Creating a Five-Star Experience

When you walk into our office, our focus is on getting you to where you need to be as fast as possible, streamlining paperwork so that there's time for true comfort and relaxation. To accomplish this, we extensively train our team on what both the patient and the doctor require so there are as few hiccups in the process as possible.

This attention to detail and process goes well beyond the evident. For instance:

- **Answering the phone right away**. This may seem obvious, but try calling your physician right now. If you're like most, your call was probably received by an automated answering service that made you pick a number, and then another number, and possibly even a third number, just so you can leave a message on an answering machine. This is not the case at our office. Our phones are answered quickly by a real person so that we can address your needs promptly.

- **Flexible Schedule**. We strive to keep flexibility in our schedule so that if the need occurs, we can see you quickly—if not the same day—at a time that's as convenient as possible.

- **Clean Spaces**. Every space associated with our office, from our parking area to the storage closet, is kept clean and in good condition. The sign for our office is easy to read from the street, so you know you're at the right place, and parking for new patients is reserved up front. The common areas and restrooms are clean and comfortable, and lightly scented so that they don't smell medical while at the same time, not overpoweringly fragrant. And there's no such thing as a worn or dirty surface in our office space. We make it a point to keep *all* glass surfaces clean, the paint fresh, and the furniture in good, clean condition.

- **Reception Desk**. Gone are the days of the non-responsive front desk person behind a tiny sliding glass window. Not only have we removed the window, but the front desk is also open and uncluttered, with a smiling front desk operator that greets you the moment you walk up. There is no waiting for someone to get off the phone and, if you were able to fill out our online forms ahead of time (sent directly to your preferred email address), there's usually no clipboard, either.

- **Waiting Room**. The waiting room is not only clean and tidy, but it's also completely devoid of old, worn, and rumpled magazines. Instead, there's a wide variety of reading material for all ages, along with a comfortably placed television (on low volume with captions, on a non-news channel that *isn't* discussing medical or dental procedures), free wi-fi, and a toy box for children with toys that are cleaned daily. We also offer chilled bottled water on request, along with other patient amenities.

- **Treatment Rooms**. We understand that the fear factor for dental offices is real and pervasive in our society. For that reason, when you walk into a treatment room, you're not going to see a lot of medical equipment sitting out. Instead, we use soft lighting, tasteful decorations, and comfortable furniture to create a more relaxed experience.

- **Our Appearance**. This may not seem like an obvious importance, but we have several rules regarding the appearance of staff and doctors in our office. Uniforms must fit correctly—neither too tight nor too loose—and dentists must wear dress clothes. Everyone, from the front desk to the doctor, must be well-groomed with tattoos covered and any body piercings removed. It may not seem like a lot, but a clean and tidy appearance—from the rooms to the staff and even the doctor—lets our clients know that we pay attention to detail, and that every detail gets professional treatment.

Perception Is Everything

A story I've often heard attributed to Don Burr, founder of the former People Express Airlines, does an excellent job of pointing out the importance of attention to every detail.

Picture yourself the last time you had to fly somewhere. Imagine you had a pretty ideal experience this time around—you checked in early online, the line for security was minimal, and your gate was conveniently close to a cafe with clean, available tables. When they called your flight, you got onboard without a hitch, found a spot for your luggage right over your seat, and got into your seat without stepping over two other people or ticking off the other passengers around you.

Everything was going brilliantly until you sat down and unfolded the tray table and there, on the surface of the table, was a huge, crusty food stain. In that moment, you suddenly became convinced that the pilot was incompetent, the wings were held on with duct tape and the engine was one decrepit shiver from bursting into flame.

Perception is everything, and if we aren't paying attention to detail, then dentists can be rest assured that their clients *are*.

Everything about your visit, from the moment you arrive, should feel like a five-star experience.

A fair number of patient satisfaction surveys suggest that while patients may like their doctor, they are most dissatisfied with the treatment they received from supporting team members. This is why our focus is a complete 180 degrees from the typical medical office experience—we spend an enormous amount of energy and effort making sure that our team is always present and aware of our clients' needs. Our staff know—and agree—that their needs come second to the needs of our patients.

From the moment you walk in the door, your experience dictates your relationship with us. Creating the best first impression requires substantial energy and effort, but if the end result is that our clients feel more comfortable, less fearful, and more respected by our doctors and staff, then it's all worth it.

Category of One

What is a "category of one" dental practice?

It's a dental practice that values the power of distinction versus the cost of blending in. It's one that goes above and beyond for its patients, creating an environment that's difficult—if not impossible—for others to duplicate.

This distinction doesn't just apply to our physical building, however. It's also found in how we treat our patients and in the services we provide. For our patients, we want to give them the kind of smile that doesn't just serve its purpose, but stands out. A "category of one" company is, at all times, a reflection of the utmost quality in all aspects of its operation and it's this type of practice that we aim to exemplify every day.

Chapter Two

WHAT IS AN UNHEALTHY SMILE COSTING YOU?

As humans go, our greatest fears are pretty specific: there's extinction, of course, as well as physical injury, loss of autonomy, separation, and ego-death.[1] If you were to put these in order, extinction would be the most powerful, followed by the others in this same order, ending in ego-death, which can also be described as "embarrassment, humiliation, or any other form of strong self-disapproval."

So, where does "fear of dentistry" fall in this? It depends on how you view a dentist visit. More than likely, it falls first under the fear of physical injury—that we'll somehow feel pain during our visit. This isn't

---

1   Karl Albrecht, "The (Only) 5 Fears We All Share," Psychology today, last modified March 22, 2012, https://www.psychologytoday.com/blog/brainsnacks/201203/the-only-5-fears-we-all-share

an uncommon fear.[2] In fact, about 75 percent of all US citizens have some degree of fear of the dentist, from mild to severe, with anywhere between 5 and 10 percent of the population experiencing true dental phobia, meaning that they'll avoid a dentist's office at all costs.[3]

What is that "cost," by the way? What is fear costing us when we won't go to the dentist because our gums bleed a little when we brush or because that one tooth is really starting to ache more often?

What are the opportunity costs of fear?

When we look back at things we've done in life that we were initially afraid of, we most often find that those fears were simply built up in our own head.

Take Geoff's story, for instance. At forty-one years old, he was only able to visit a dentist under IV sedation, and had been that way for at least twenty-five years. For Geoff, this severely limited the dentists he could go to, and meant that he only saw them when something was wrong. In this particular case, he arrived at a dental hospital with tooth pain and an examination showed that he had no less than three teeth that needed to come out. After he had them extracted under sedation, however, Geoff was able to undergo therapy that allowed him to slowly ease into a dental office and eventually have a tooth restored and two cavities filled with just a local anesthetic; with no IV and fully conscious.[4]

---

2   Keep in mind that while the statistics are relatively US specific, Canadian statistics are relatively close in comparison.

3   Peter Milgrom, Philip Weinstein, and Tracy Getz, *Treating Fearful Dental Patients: A Patient Management Handbook, 2nd Edition* (Seattle, WA: University of Washington, Cont, 1995)

4   K.I. Wilson and J.G. Davies, "A joint approach to treating dental phobics between community dental services and specialist psychotherapy services – a single case report," *British Dental Journal* 190, no. 8 (April 2001): 431–2, https://doi.org/10.1038/sj.bdj.4800993a

If Geoff had been able to deal with his fear earlier in life and simply visited his dentist regularly, it's likely he never would have needed such extensive work done. That is, in a nutshell, a whole bunch of opportunity costs—by choosing to let fear keep him from the dentist, it cost him twenty-five years of proactive dental visits, tooth pain from lack of treatment, dental damage, and likely the impact to his self-esteem for a quarter of a century because of a poor smile.

When you think back on your own life, it's likely there are more than a few instances where you had to walk through your fear instead of backing away from it—and you probably found out that you'd made it a lot more frightening in your own head than it was in actuality.

Are Bad Teeth Telling Your Life Story?

Your smile tells your life story faster than any other means known to humanity. First impressions are made in milliseconds, and while research is still trying to pinpoint all the details of how we're able to assess people so quickly, we do know that common facial features play an incredible role in other people's initial—and lasting—perception of you.

"A first glance at a person's face often leaves a lasting impression," writes psychologist Vivian Diller in a July 2012 article for *Psychology Today*. "Facial features are more often remembered following initial interactions than people's bodies or even their personality traits."

Diller goes on to note several conclusions that people make based on their first impression of our eyes, nose, skin, and hair, as well as our smile and our teeth, all of which are viewed and assessed in less than a second.

"A person's smile is the feature that elicits the most immediate and positive reaction from others," Diller states. "People who have a spontaneous and natural smile ... send an inviting message to others. It says 'come join me, talk to me.'" An unsmiling face, however, "can say, 'I'm not interested.' A frown says, 'go away.'"

Teeth, too, leave a strong impression. "While we may not all have dazzling straight pearly whites, having good oral hygiene goes along with the positive impact that a great smile brings," writes Diller. "Severely crooked or yellowing teeth can imply you are a smoker or heavy drinker. Mottled teeth can reflect certain illnesses, poor nutrition, or an eating disorder. Fresh and bright teeth generally suggest that you are someone with a healthy lifestyle and good grooming habits."

Photogenic or Not, Good Teeth Matter

Good teeth are a hot topic on the acting website Backstage.com. In an article titled "Nothing But the Tooth," actors speak to how improvements to their smiles made significant differences in their careers.

"Before I got my teeth whitened, they [casting directors] made comments suggesting that I was not going to be on TV," said actor Sonora Chase. "That has changed."

Actor Jessica Delfino also shared that a quality veneer made all the difference in her performing career, taking her from being self-conscious about a poorly repaired front tooth to having the confidence to take on the "perfection-loving media."

According to Dr. Michelle Callahan, "Whether we like it or not, we are often judged by our appearance...your smile has more of an effect on what others perceive about you than you think."

In a perception study conducted by marketing research firm Kelton, more than a thousand participants were asked to give their honest opinion on the people in a variety of images, and what they found was that those with straight teeth appeared to have more desirable qualities than those with crooked teeth, including the snap judgment that they were "happy" and "professionally successful."

In comparison to people with crooked teeth, the perception study also noted that Americans perceive those with straight teeth as being:

- 45 percent more likely to get a job
- 58 percent more successful
- 57 percent more likely to get a date
- 47 percent more likely to be viewed as healthy

Additionally, close to three in five Americans would rather have a nice smile than clear skin, and 87 percent would give up something for a year if it meant having a nice smile for the rest of their life.

So what story is your smile telling others? And just as importantly, how is that story affecting your *life story* going forward?

"Research clearly shows that having decayed or missing teeth has a strong negative impact on self-esteem," notes psychologist Daniel W. McNeil, PhD. "It also has an impact on employability."[5]

---

5   Rebecca A. Clay, "Drilling down on dental fears," *Monitor on Psychology* 47, no. 3 (March 2016): 60, http://www.apa.org/monitor/2016/03/dental-fears.aspx

Bad Teeth, No Job

When the American Dental Association took a look at oral health and well-being in the United States in 2015, it uncovered some alarming statistics. Young adults were almost neck-and-neck with low income adults in agreeing that "the appearance of my mouth and teeth affects my ability to interview for a job," and one in four adults avoid smiling due to the condition of their mouth and teeth. Judging by what we just learned from psychologist Vivian Diller, this means that a quarter of adults are unintentionally hurting the first impression they give others just because they're too embarrassed to smile.

For a case in point, just look at the story of "Shelly" as reported by the Deseret News in Salt Lake City, Utah.

In 2012, a counseling office in Salt Lake City was looking for a front desk employee and while they were getting plenty of applicants, none met all of their specific qualifications. Then, Shelly arrived at the office as a temp. A thirty-five-year-old mother of three, she was reportedly "pleasant to work with, competent, and kind to the patients." In fact, another front desk employee urged leadership to hire Shelly on permanently. Yet, when her temp position ended, the company chose not to bring her on.

When asked why Shelly wasn't hired, employees were apparently told that it was because she had bucked, crooked teeth.

"He [the office manager] said it wasn't the image we wanted to project at our clinic," said one of the front desk employees.[6]

---

6   Mercedes White, "No teeth means no job," Deseret News, last modified December 27, 2012, https://www.deseretnews.com/article/865569512/No-teeth-means-no-job-How-poor-oral-health-impacts-job-prospects.html

Image is the New Communication

Communication is becoming more and more image-focused, with social media reflecting this through a massive uptick in video messaging. As of 2017, more than 70 percent of Gen-Z (those born after 1995) spent more than three hours a day watching videos online, and their social platforms of choice, such as SnapChat and Whisper, are almost solely image and video-based.[7]

While most employers aren't as obvious about their motivations in hiring or not hiring certain individuals, you can be certain that a good smile is going to play a big part in other people's first and ongoing impression of you: a factor that a woman in California was well aware of as she sat outside of a state dental clinic overnight.

At fifty-three years old, Patty knew she needed dental work if she was going to land a job. As she waited outside of the clinic, she told an NBC news reporter about her five broken teeth, three cavities and gum abscess, and how the pain was only part of the reason she was there—she knew the condition of her teeth was an important part of the hiring process.

"I really don't smile a lot," she told the reporter. "I know that when you have a job, you want to have a pleasant attitude and you've got to smile and be friendly."

The report went on to quote Dr. Susan Hyde, a dentist and population scientist at the University of California in San Francisco,

---

7   Nelson Granados, "Gen Z Media Consumption: It's A Lifestyle, Not Just Entertainment," Media & Entertainment, Forbes, last modified June 20, 2017,
    https://www.forbes.com/sites/nelsongranados/2017/06/20/gen-z-media-consumption-its-a-lifestyle-not-just-entertainment/

"If you want to portray someone as being wicked, they have missing front teeth. If they're ignorant, they have buck teeth. Even from a very early age, we associate how one presents their oral health with all kinds of biases that reflect some of the social biases that we have."

Dr. Lindsey Robinson, dentist and president of the California Dental Association, added, "Customer service jobs, good entry-level jobs … they're not available to people who have lost the basic ability to smile, to function, to chew properly."[8]

But the chain of consequences resulting from bad teeth doesn't stop here. Poor dental health can also affect your immediate health, and apart from making it difficult to work when you're not feeling well, it can affect your long-term wellbeing and can even result in death.

A Heart Attack … and Diabetes, Stroke, and Cardiovascular Disease … Waiting to Happen

In 2007, a twelve-year-old boy in Washington, D.C. died from a toothache. It was a combination of unfortunate circumstances that led to the tragic event, but ultimately, what could have been an $80 routine extraction ended up costing him his life. His family paid close to $250,000 in medical care, including brain surgery in an attempt to save the boy from the infection that had spread from a tooth abscess into his brain.[9]

---

8   Jonel Aleccia, "Bad teeth, broken dreams: Lack of dental care keeps many out of jobs," NBC News, last modified June 12, 2013, https://www.nbcnews.com/feature/in-plain-sight/bad-teeth-broken-dreams-lack-dental-care-keeps-many-out-v18906511

9   Mary Otto, "For Want of a Dentist," Washington Post, last modified February 28, 2007, http://www.washingtonpost.com/wp-dyn/content/article/2007/02/27/AR2007022702116.html

This is an extreme instance, but the fact is that bacteria, which accumulate quickly in the mouth as they feed on the food particles surrounding un-brushed teeth, have instant access to the bloodstream through the inflamed gums that occur with periodontal disease. These bacteria don't go through any filtering process, either, as they would if they entered the body through the lungs, stomach, ears or nose. In other words, inflammation, the gaps created by a receding gum line, and other untreated dental conditions, are akin to having an un-bandaged open wound on your body. Those bacteria can jump right in and start wreaking havoc, which is why researchers are discovering that there are more diseases than just the obvious ones associated with poor dental health.

The following links between poor dental health and disease are described in depth by the National Institute of Health's report "Oral Health in America: A Report of the Surgeon General": https://www. nidcr.nih.gov/DataStatistics/SurgeonGeneral/sgr/home.htm

- **COPD**. COPD, or chronic obstructive pulmonary disease, is caused by chronic bronchitis, emphysema, or recurring respiratory infection, and has been associated with periodontal disease due to bacterial pneumonia living in the mouth and making its way into the airway.

- **Diabetes**. Periodontitis has been linked to diabetes—both types 1 and 2—so often that it's now being referred to as one of the main complications of diabetes. Reports have suggested that it's a two-way street for these diseases, as well—that diabetics are more likely to get periodontal disease, and periodontal disease may have a negative impact on glycemic control.

- ***Heart Disease and Stroke***. Evidence is continuing to grow on the relationship between infectious agents and systemic diseases, with certain bacteria that thrive in dental infections being identified as potentially linked to heart disease. For example, as we said earlier, bacteria or viruses in the mouth can get directly into the blood stream, where they can cause inflammation, blood clots, and narrowing of the arteries.

- ***Preterm Birth and Low Birth Weight***. Bacterial infection in the mouth may contribute to adverse pregnancy outcomes, as the harmful bacteria and other toxins created by the infection can get into the blood, cross the placenta, and harm the fetus. Additionally, the reaction of the mother's immune system to the infection could directly or indirectly interfere with growth and/or delivery.

This Isn't Just About Teeth—It's About the Rest of Your Life

This book isn't about promoting dentistry. It's about helping you discover the long-term opportunity costs of fear and the importance of being proactive about the health of your smile.

The first step is understanding the importance of a healthy mouth, which you should have a better idea of after reading this book. The next step? Understanding that when you're not healthy, you're not living at your full potential.

Chapter Three

UNLEASHING HUMAN POTENTIAL

At the age of fourteen, Susan still remembers the conversation that took place between her dentist and her parents, when her dentist first urged them to take her to an orthodontist. There was some medical terminology batted about, but one line stuck with her so clearly that she can still hear her dentist saying it today; "If you don't do something now, we'll probably have to break her jaw when she's older."

If she hadn't heard her dentist say that, she might have fussed a little more about the braces her orthodontist fitted her with, but instead she took it all in stride and even switched out her bracket bands to reflect the holidays as they went by. A little over a year later, the braces came off and everyone in the office "ooh"ed and "ahh"ed over her beautiful smile.

Fast forward to a little over two decades later and thirty-seven-year-old Susan couldn't quite remember when she stopped wearing her retainer, though she was sure it was within a year or two after getting her braces off, and certainly before she went to college. Consequently, her teeth had drifted to the point where she could noticeably tell a difference in how they sat in her mouth.

One of the issues people face when it comes to maintaining a healthy smile is the lack of clarity around the natural aging process and its impact on your teeth. Orthodontic relapse is a condition that a lot of post-braces patients fall victim to, and one that we see in the dental office pretty frequently. The issue is that people rarely understand the importance of wearing a retainer and the fact that time and other dental conditions down the road can all affect the hard work that your doctors put into that straight smile so many years ago.

After braces, teeth need at least one year to stabilize and get used to their new positions in the jaw. This is when retainer wear is at its most important—to protect the teeth from relapsing into their former positions and allow them time to solidify in their new positions in the jaws. If a retainer isn't worn, or is worn infrequently, during this time, the teeth may shift and if the patient doesn't visit her dentist, she may not notice that shift for some time.

Even if a retainer is worn for at least a year, after the patient stops wearing it, the teeth once again fall victim to outside—and inside—influences. Teeth grinding, for instance, can place strain on the teeth of the upper jaw, and tooth loss can cause the remaining teeth to drift into the vacant spot. Internal influences could be genetics, which can prompt your teeth to shift, for instance, or gum disease can cause the structure to weaken.

And then there's simply the age factor. As we age, pressures on the teeth can cause them to shift, so even if Susan did wear her retainer for a few years after braces, twenty years is a long time for teeth to react to any influences, internal or external.

In neglecting her teeth, Susan neglected the potential that straight teeth could have resulted in. Apart from generally giving her a healthier appearance, straight teeth also create a healthier mouth in actuality—with straight teeth, there are fewer places for food and bacteria to hide, making it easier to brush. And straight teeth also make chewing easier, which means less strain on the jaw, which means avoiding jaw joint issues down the road.

It's like the old adage "for want of a nail, the kingdom was lost." By not maintaining a healthy smile and being proactive about it, we open the gates to numerous problems down the road. For Susan, drifting teeth meant that they were sitting in less-than-ideal positions in her mouth, making them harder to brush, which meant more bacterial buildup. And more bacterial buildup can cause inflammation of the gums. Inflammation leads to gingivitis, gingivitis leads to periodontal disease and periodontal disease leads to … well, you read the last chapter, right? It could potentially lead to anything from heart disease to death.

All for the want of proactive, preventative dental care.

Hitting the Reset Button On Your Smile

Unlike many things in life, you have the option of hitting the reset button on your smile. It doesn't matter if you've smoked your whole life or if illegal drug use has caused most of your teeth to rot out—whatever you've done, technology and advancements in dental science have made it possible to rebuild just about any smile.

We live in a world today where photos are uploaded by the billions every single day. In 2014, for instance, it was estimated that every two minutes, the same number of photos were uploaded to the Internet as existed in the world one hundred and fifty years ago. This is a world where you can no longer hide your smile.[10] The camera is on you constantly and whether or not you realize it, it's having an impact on the course of your life. People make snap judgments based on the images they see of you, and based on their first 0.1 seconds of interacting with you. You're regularly being assessed in situations and under circumstances where you cannot speak for yourself—your image is doing all of the talking.

I'm aware this probably sounds superficial, but regardless of our better efforts, we're still a superficial species. Our instincts still react the same way they did eons ago—an attractive smile still triggers the selection of a mate. It still inclines us to like or trust someone more. Genuine smiles, also called Duchenne smiles—the ones that get you to use those little muscles around your eyes—also signal to others that you're focusing on just them, which in turn encourages them to cooperate with you.[11]

At the same time, the way you feel about your smile also influences your own perception of self. Your self-concept is determined, many times, by the way you look at yourself in the mirror. Do you smile at yourself from ear to ear or do you frown in an effort to conceal your imperfect grin? That perception lives with you and reflects outward, whether you realize it or not, affecting not only your own happiness, but the happiness you could be generating in others.

---

10   Rose Eveleth, "How Many Photographs of You Are Out There In The World?" The Atlantic, last modified November 2, 2015, https://www.theatlantic.com/technology/archive/2015/11/how-many-photographs-of-you-are-out-there-in-the-world/413389/

11   Gil Greengross, "Want to Increase Trust in Others? Just Smile," Psychology Today, last modified April 30, 2015, https://www.psychologytoday.com/blog/humor-sapiens/201504/want-increase-trust-in-others-just-smile-0

There is no doubt that a bright and vibrant smile can do more to drive happiness in someone's life than you would think on the surface. When you think about it, what are the things you could do in life that will ultimately drive happiness? Most likely, the majority of those things can be traced back to your ability to smile.

What Makes Us Happy?

Research shows that around 40 percent of our own happiness is under our control. So what can you do to make yourself happier - and how do those behaviors relate to your smile?

1. Strong relationships with people you trust

2. Good income / paying bills without stress

3. Taking the time to think about the good things in life

4. Performing voluntary acts of kindness

5. Exercising

6. Living life instead of buying things

7. Living in the moment - mindful meditation

8. Time with friends

Unleashing Human Potential

A lot of people ask me what I do professionally, and when I tell them that I'm a dentist, the typical reaction is, "Oh, you fix teeth."

If only it were that simple.

One of the big reasons I got into dentistry was because I realized the power that a confident smile can give someone. And I realized that when people have a smile they can be proud of, they show it a lot more.

I found that the more people smiled, the more confident they were and the easier it was for them to speak and communicate. These people had a higher self-image, and a better self-concept. And believe it or not, I found that the more people smiled, the more career and professional success they experienced and the more productive relationships they had.

So when people jump straight to "you pull teeth" once I tell them I'm a dentist—well, it's not nearly that simple. What I and everyone else in our office are in the business of doing is unleashing human potential. We help our patients regain their ability to smile, and by doing so, we also help them acquire confidence, capability, and allow them to be more ready to take on the opportunities in the world and achieve great success for themselves and for their families in the process.

Case Study: What a Yearbook Smiles Tells Us

Over the course of thirty years, Drs. LeeAnne Harker and Dacher Keltner followed the lives of one hundred women after graduating from college to determine if a positive emotional expression in their yearbook photo was linked to their life outcomes.

During the study, Harker and Keltner, along with their research team, contacted the women in the study at ages twenty-one, twenty-seven, forty-three, and fifty-two, asking them various questions about marriage, family, and work, among other topics. What they found was that "over time, women who expressed more positive emotion in their yearbook pictures became more organized, mentally focused, and achievement oriented, and less susceptible to repeated and prolonged experiences of negative affect." In addition, they confirmed theories that "individual differences in positive emotional expression were linked to personal stability and development across adulthood, the impressions and reactions from other people, and the marital satisfaction and well-being up to thirty years later, " adding that, "People photograph each other with casual and remarkable frequency, usually unaware that each snapshot may capture as much about the future as it does the passing emotions of the moment."[12]

Overcoming Fear with Practice

Now that you understand the fear, the consequences, and the motivation of a healthy mouth, let me share with you how we're working to change the dental experience forever. The first and most important step is education—knowing the *why* behind regular visits to the dentist—but the next is on me and my team, which is to make those visits the absolute best they can possibly be. Doctors can't afford to continue with the old-fashioned model of making patients wait on

---

12   LeeAnne Harker and Dacher Keltner, "Expressions of Positive Emotion in Women's College Yearbook Pictures and Their Relationship to Personality and Life Outcomes Across Adulthood," *Journal of Personality and Social Psychology* 80, no. 1 (January 2001): 112–124, https://doi.org/10.1037/0022-3514.80.1.112

them. Today, it's the complete opposite. Only those doctors that are willing to put their patients front and center—to cater to *their* needs instead of the other way around—are the ones that are going to survive. And we intend to do more than survive—we intend to make your needs our number one priority, and in doing so, become *your* number one dentist.

Chapter Four

BEST TEAM IN TOWN

Over the years, I've spent a lot of time developing clinical skills, attending advanced training courses and doing everything I could think of to offer my patients the best and most up-to-date care possible. What I was missing, however, was the understanding that my team is the most impactful reflection of my ability. I could go through all the training in the world, but if lackadaisical staff members are treating my patients poorly, that knowledge and experience would never counterbalance that negative first impression.

Today, I understand that we have to stay at the highest possible level of clinical skills, training, and technology, not only to keep up with the rapidly evolving pace of dental technology, but to also provide our patients with the absolute highest quality of service.

The "best team in town" concept is our belief that we should not only have the most competent clinical team on the floor, but also a team that is present in all situations and circumstances, has been trained to stay focused on the patient, and a team that will never compromise on their work. This means that everything from the way appointments are scheduled when you call to how you're greeted when you walk in the door, how you're escorted to the treatment room, and even how you are communicated with should be top-notch and focused only on you.

It's Not a Job, It's a Career

One of our primary goals is to turn each role at our office into a career. This means reinforcing each team member's overall commitment to the practice and the patient, connecting them to the mission of our organization and encouraging them to apply our core values both personally and professionally.

Our Core Values

Ethical, Hard Working, Accountable, Professional, Positive, Adaptable, Proactive, Engaged

---

Through modeling core values, it's our hope that our staff will have more of a positive impact simply through the behaviors they exhibit, particularly when interacting with patients and with each other.

In other areas, we strive to make a positive impact by providing our staff with the best training, coached in the understanding that we expect from them the highest level of commitment and expectation. As a patient, we want you to understand that we're taking all of these steps to dramatically improve your experience. Our training both in clinical skills and continuing education are not just a "bare minimum" effort, but are undertaken in order to stay ahead of the curve and at the top of our game.

One of these efforts ties directly into our desire to be a Patient-Centric office, which is engendering in our staff—and particularly our hygienists—the desire to not just treat the patient, but to be their Oral Health Advocate.

Consider the following feedback we received from a hygienist shortly after going through patient-centric training:

The Honest Truth: *A statement from a Veteran Hygienist*

The biggest problem that I see with other hygienists in other offices is that they aren't stepping up to the plate to be their patients' Oral Healthcare Advocate … not just a hygienist. I'm not pointing fingers—I've been in those shoes.

I used to tell a patient what they needed to know about a procedure, and when they showed the slightest pushback, I would give up. I didn't know how to handle their irritation, their impatience, and their questions about financing, but I realized that was *my fault*. And because I didn't know how to communicate how big of an impact this decision was going to have on their life, they didn't get the care that they deserved.

As hygienists, if we don't step up for the patient, then we are the ones that are keeping a problem alive that has existed in the dental industry for way too long.

I still remember the day that this was made real to me. I was standing in the break room, drinking coffee and complaining about the training session that I and the other staff members had to take that day. We walked into the training room, all of us still highly skeptical. But then, the trainer started talking, and the truth of what she said hit me in the stomach. How she described the importance of advocating for our patients changed the way I looked at my career forever. From that day on, I knew I couldn't keep doing things the same way. I was no longer an "oral janitor" but an Oral Healthcare Advocate. My life's purpose is to give my patients healthier smiles and healthier lives, and to get as many other people to join me as possible. I'm telling you, I'm ready to start a revolution.

What I do is not just a nine-to-five job. It's not just a paycheck. Being a hygienist is our chance to serve—and to save lives. During my training, I realized that, as Oral Healthcare Advocates, we're literally the only people in our patient's lives that are aware of their oral health, so we can't be afraid to tell them what they need to do. Our patients trust us 100 percent to tell them what treatment is the best possible one for them.

As a hygienist, if you know that a procedure will benefit your patient, but you don't give 100 percent effort in educating them on it, then you are doing that patient a serious disservice. They don't know what you do, but they want to understand and they won't know what to ask unless you give them as much information as you can.

That's just the honest truth. If you're doing any less, then you aren't fulfilling your duties as a healthcare provider. It isn't that you have bad intentions if you don't—none of us do! Since becoming a hygienist, I've realized that the people in this industry are some of the warmest, most caring individuals I've ever met. But this epidemic of apathy has to stop. Some hygienists are out there doing the bare minimum of service rather than consistently over-delivering to their patients—being reactive instead of proactive about their treatment. I know that we can do better than that.

During training, our team learned to refocus on what each patient truly needs, and we made it our mission to give him or her the best solution. I now feel empowered to give my patients a healthier life and to take responsibility for that patient like I would a member of my own family.

Continuing Education

In addition to standard and continuing education, our staff may be participating in upward of one hundred hours of training per year on subjects directly related to the customer experience, such as the oral healthcare advocate training the hygienist spoke to earlier.

Our focus is on having a consistent process for everything from the front desk to the hygienists, to dental assistants, to the doctors in the practice. It's these processes that allow us to work with the other professionals in our office so that every patient receives the same, consistent quality of care.

Our Office is a "No Judgment" Zone

Let's address the elephant in the room right now—people judge. They judge us by our appearance, by the clothes we wear, by our opinions, even by the way we cut our hair. That may be able to slip under the radar at other establishments, but that attitude of judgment is left at the door at our office. If any one of our employees walks in with a judgmental chip on their shoulder, then that's the day they lose their job.

We do *not* judge anyone who comes to us. We do not allow any unchecked personal opinions from our team members drive how you are treated. We don't treat you differently based on what type of insurance you have or if you don't have insurance—we're simply interested in understanding what it is you need or want to have done, making sure you're comfortable, and providing you with what you need.

As a doctor, we want our patients to understand that this is not a normal commitment, but it is one that I believe is key to the relationship we share with our patients and the reason why our number one source for new patients today is referrals from existing ones.

Chapter Five

STEWARD OF YOUR SMILE

Let me ask you a question—have you ever worn down your tires and gotten a flat?

If so, what did you do? Did you go to the mechanic and ask for a patch, or did you get a new tire?

A lot of us have opted for the patch—even when the tires are so worn they're practically bald because we tell ourselves that we just can't afford new tires right then. When that happens, however, what do we end up doing? Eventually we have get that new tire, but we're spending more for it because we've had to pay for the patch and any other damage that happened to the car from running on bald tires until we bought new ones.

More often than not, we do more damage and end up costing ourselves more when we choose to "patch" instead of truly repair.

It's the very same situation with your smile. Your teeth bear much of the brunt of your lifestyle. If you enjoy acidic beverages such as coffee, wine or energy drinks, then that enamel is getting worn down every day. If your diet is high in sugar, then your teeth are constantly being bombarded by bacteria, and that's even if you're brushing the recommended two times a day (which a staggering one in five people *do not* do).

Taking care of your mouth is more than just brushing—there's a lot more that goes into it, and yet so few of us are on the preventative side of smile care. For instance, tell me—do your gums bleed when you brush? Do you ever notice a little bit of a gap between your gum and your tooth when you feel around your teeth with your tongue? Or is there buildup on a tooth or two that you just can't get off with brushing?

All of these conditions—gingivitis, receding gum line, and plaque buildup, respectively—are signs you need to see your dentist as soon as possible, and yet so many of us ignore these kinds of issues until they start to hurt. And by then, the conditions have likely progressed to point where more involved treatments may be necessary.

It's the strangest thing! We could go see the dentist every six months, get our teeth cleaned, floss regularly, and let the dentist take care of minor cavities as they occur, or we could do as more than a third of Americans do and just not go to the dentist until those preventative conditions become a severe problem.[13]

Acidic and sugary drinks and snacks aren't the only challenges that our teeth face on a regular basis. There's also the impact of stress on teeth—grinding (also called "bruxism") is associated with anxiety

---

13   Lecia Bushak, "Oral Health Isn't Much Of Americans' Concern, Poll Finds: One-Third Didn't See The Dentist Last Year," Medical Daily, last modified April 29, 2014, http://www.medicaldaily.com/oral-health-isnt-much-americans-concern-poll-finds-one-third-didnt-see-dentist-last-year-279468

and depression, and can cause you to wear away your enamel and expose the dentin, which is much softer than the enamel and can lead to sensitivity and cavities.[14] It could even cause your teeth to crack and, over the long-term, it can lead to complications with your jaw joint (also called the "TMJ" or temporomandibular joint) and may even cause facial muscles to become enlarged from overuse, potentially blocking your salivary glands, which then can lead to inflammation, pain, and dry mouth … which leads to more cavities, and so on.[15]

We define stewardship as "protecting and growing the owner's assets with fierce intensity." Therefore, taking stewardship of your smile is about recognizing that your health is a valuable belonging, and taking those preventative measures is paramount to maintaining your oral health so you never reach the point of paying $10,000 for a repair that could have been a minor fix if you'd seen your dentist on a regular basis.

When you do run into those repairs, though, stewardship is also about making the best choice for your smile rather than the cheapest one. Remember the tires analogy? Patching your problem ultimately ends up costing you more than getting it right the first time. And as your dentist, I never want to encourage you to just patch something five or six times when we can eliminate the problem once and for all.

---

14   Angelina R. Sutin et al., "Teeth grinding: Is Emotional Stability related to bruxism?" *Journal of Research in Personality 44*, no. 3 (June 2010): 402–405, https://doi.org/10.1016/j.jrp.2010.03.006

15   Donna Pleis, "Teeth Clenching And Grinding Can Affect Your Dental Health," Bruxism, Colgate, last modified, http://www.colgate.com/en/us/oc/oral-health/conditions/bruxism/article/teeth-clenching-and-grinding-can-affect-your-dental-health-1114

Why We Don't Care Who Your Insurance Carrier Is

When it comes to your health and your smile, my first thought is always going to be "What's the right thing to do here?" It's about what we can do to protect you and help you grow and live a full and happy life. If a close relative comes to me with a dental condition, for instance, I'm not going to tell her how to patch it for now—I'm going to tell her how to fix it for the long-term. And the same goes with my patients—I don't want to recommend temporary repair when you will be far better served in the long-term by fixing it right the first time.

This is why we don't care who your insurance carrier is. Ultimately, your insurance is never going to give you everything you need. We accept it, but if it costs more, then we'll find a way to make it work. Financing is readily available and there are ways to make it affordable. But insurance should never be the deciding factor. We are taking care of *you and your family*, not your checkbook, and how well you take care of your mouth impacts every aspect of your life from the day you're born and will follow you to the grave.

What Is the Cost of Neglecting Your Dental Health?

Health is an interesting value. It's something we all need and yet, it's not something we can purchase. We can't walk into a gym and say, "Okay, I'll take two well-defined biceps, a washboard stomach and a set of toned glutes. How much will that be?" Instead, we have to work hard to produce and maintain a healthy body on our own.

It takes time and it takes discipline, but for the sake of our overall health, it's worth it.

When we say "worth it," however, what do we mean? There's the personal, innate worth, of course—the cost of time and effort put into brushing our teeth or hitting the gym are "worth" it when it leaves us feeling healthier. But there are also physical financial benefits to good health, as well.

One economics researcher, Michael Grossman put it well when he described human behavior regarding health: "Individuals inherit an initial stock of health that … can be increased by investment," adding that "Individuals 'choose' their length of life" when investments are made through direct inputs into that stock, such as medical care, diet, exercise, and recreation.

If you really enjoy reading into the process of creating economic models, then you should certainly check out Grossman's paper "On the Concept of Health Capital and the Demand for Health." Otherwise, I'll just get right to one of his conclusions, which is that when we take stock of our life (or, in this case, look at it like investing in stock), we can predict that the more educated people are about the benefits of good health, including longevity, the more proactive they'll be about obtaining it.[16]

Consider the following study conducted by a group in Scotland, who set out to determine whether or not a country-wide nursery toothbrushing program was not only making a difference in the longer term dental health of children, but if it was also saving money on dental costs down the road. Specifically, the study looked at the cost savings from improvements in the dental health of five year olds

---

16 Michael Grossman, "On the Concept of Health Capital and the Demand for Health," *Journal of Political Economy* 80, no. 2 (April 1972): 223–255, https://doi.org/10.1086/259880

through the avoidance of needing extractions, fillings, or other treatments due to decay.

The first step was determining the complete costs for filling or extracting a decayed primary tooth, and then on average, how many of those dental treatments were conducted over a ten-year period.

They found that not only did the dental treatments for five year olds decrease over time once the toothbrushing program was initiated, but by the program's eighth year, the expected financial savings alone were two and a half times the cost of the program.[17]

How, then, can we be proactive about dental health? With two simple initial investments:

1. Brushing and flossing at least twice a day

2. Visiting your dentist at least twice a year.

That's all the investment you need to make on a stock that can have incredibly rewarding returns.

Opportunity Costs of Dental Health

Essentially, an opportunity cost is the choice that you give up when you make a decision. That is, when given the choice between "gum" and "a mint" and you choose "a mint," the opportunity cost is the gum.

When you expand on that idea, "opportunity cost" not only stands for the loss of one choice in preference of another, it also represents the long-term consequences of your choice.

If we stick with the gum/mint choice, for instance, by choosing the mint, we could, say, miss out on the longer-term benefit of

---

17   Yulia Anopa et al., "Improving Child Oral Health: Cost Analysis of a National Nursery Toothbrushing Programme," *PLoS ONE* 10, no. 8 (August 2015), http://doi.org/10.1371/journal.pone.0136211

chewing gum. If the gum was sugarless and the mint was not, we'd be taking a hit on calorie intake by choosing the mint (as well as doing just that much more potential damage to the teeth thanks to that extended sugar exposure). Extrapolate that even further and maybe chewing gum could have kept us from thinking about eating a snack—but by taking the mint, we experienced a sugar spike and now we're eating a burrito at 2:30 p.m. instead of taking a walk, and by the end of the week, we've gained three pounds.

Opportunity Cost of Dental Health

OPTIONS: *brush and floss teeth everyday* **OR** *don't brush and floss teeth everyday*

CHOICE: *don't brush and floss teeth everyday*

WHY? *because I don't have time*

COST: *new implants to replace the rotten ones $3,000 to $6,000 per tooth*

Opportunity costs can be subjective, but they can also be quite objective and practical. In this case, consider the opportunity cost of deciding not to brush and floss every day.

The mouth is the perfect breeding ground for bacteria, and not just one type, either—there are close to four hundred different species of microorganisms, mostly bacteria, living on every filmy surface and in every hard-to-brush crevice.

According to dental researcher Sigmund Socransky, "In a clean mouth, one thousand to one hundred thousand bacteria live on each tooth surface. A person who doesn't have a terribly clean mouth can have 100 million to one billion bacteria growing on each tooth."[18]

While a good amount of those bacteria and microorganisms are beneficial, helping to fight off disease-carrying microorganisms that try to enter the body through the mouth, the oral cavity can also house harmful bacteria that, if not brushed away, can eventually irritate the gums, causing gingivitis, which evolves into periodontal disease. At this point, some of the most direct results of poor dental health may occur, including bad breath (otherwise known as halitosis) and tooth loss.

I discussed several of the following related conditions in an earlier chapter, but they're important enough to bring up again as the stewardship of your dental health can quite literally mean the difference between life and death. Those open, bleeding gums provide instant access to the bloodstream, where their presence has been linked to conditions such as:

- **Dementia**: researchers following more than five thousand people for eighteen years found that those "who reported not brushing their teeth daily had a 22 percent to 65 percent greater risk of dementia than those who brushed three times a day." Another, smaller study on Alzheimer's has noted that the brains of those with the disease exhibited more bacteria associated with gum disease than those without the mental illness.

- **Endocarditis**: bacterial infection of the lining of the heart and its valves, causing inflammation and infection

---

18   Jane E. Stevens, "Oral Ecology," MIT Technolgy Review, last modified January 1, 1997, https://www.technologyreview.com/s/400012/oral-ecology/

- *Heart disease*: wherein harmful bacteria make their way directly to the heart

- *Stroke*: bacteria-related inflammation of arterial walls and blood clotting can cause the arteries to narrow and lead to stroke

- *Rheumatoid arthritis*: periodontal disease can increase the pain caused by this disease

- *Lung disease*: both pneumonia and chronic obstructive pulmonary disorder (COPD) can be worsened by harmful bacteria making its way from the mouth to the lungs

- *Brain Abscess*: as noted earlier in the case of the twelve-year-old who died from a decayed tooth-related brain abscess, bacterial infections of the mouth can be life-threatening if left untreated. [19]

It only takes about three days of not brushing for detrimental conditions to form. Once you pass seventy-two hours, the volume of bacteria will have reached the point where they're producing enough acid to carve holes in tooth enamel, and plaque may have solidified to the point where it becomes difficult, if not impossible, to remove without professional intervention.[20]

What, then, is the opportunity cost of choosing not to brush and floss your teeth at least twice a day? It could be the cost of a filling, an implant, dentures, your overall health and even, your life.

---

19 Lauren F. Friedman, "13 Awful Things That Happen If You Don't Brush And Floss Your Teeth," Business Insider, last modified February 14, 2014, http://www.businessinsider.com/what-happens-if-you-dont-brush-and-floss-your-teeth-2014-2

20 Jane E. Stevens, "Oral Ecology," MIT Technolgy Review, last modified January 1, 1997, https://www.technologyreview.com/s/400012/oral-ecology/

Steward of your Smile

In our office, we adhere to the stewardship model, which is to protect you, to help you make good decisions and to help you grow as a person through the things that we can have an impact on.

When it comes to treatment, first and foremost, we believe in being good stewards of our patients, their time, their financial resources, and all of the transactions that occur in our business, which means helping our patients steward over their decisions in a meaningful and productive way. This is because we've found that many non-patient-centric offices will guide their treatment path based upon what they think the ability of the patient is to pay. This is simply *not* the philosophy that we use.

Instead, we treat you as a person and make recommendations to you as though you're a member of our family and allow you to ultimately make the decision that's right for you. We believe in providing you with the best recommendation for your condition, and the only way to do that is to leave the question of funding out of the picture.

As I pointed out earlier, there are times when budgets require people to patch something, be it a leak in a pipe, a hole in a weak roof, or a tire. But when we think about that decision over the long run, patching is pretty much a guaranteed way to have the problem return, and likely in a worse way than the first time around. This is why we like to give patients the option to fix things correctly the first time since it winds up being more cost effective and better for the patient overall.

Take the leaking pipe, for example. Patched, it may work a little while longer, but when it starts to leak again, that leak will likely go unchecked for a certain period of time and eventually cause more damage than it did when it was patched. The cost then ends up being the cost of fixing the problem correctly and repairing the damage done in the meantime. So which is the more cost-effective solution?

Convenient Financial Arrangements

When we consider the financial part of any visit to our office, we always approach it with these words in mind: flexible and without fear. We don't want to avoid discussing it—it's something we'll need to talk about anyway, so why not get it out there? But we don't want it to be awkward or to become a barrier to working with us. For these reasons, we offer multiple options for patient financing, including flexible payment plans.

In all cases, we like to provide our patients with options because there are times when we need to patch, but we always make sure to provide all of the information for the appropriate fix, as well, and discuss financial options if the budget is a problem. Above all, it's important to us that we educate our patients on the conditions resulting from either decision, including the consequences of patching versus fixing something correctly. Ultimately, the choice is in the patient's hands inside of our practice.

Chapter Six

THE POWER OF A FREE DAY OF DENTISTRY

One of the foundations of our practice is financial stewardship, and an important part of that is committing to living off of less than you earn, and giving a portion of what we make to the community.

We do this through several means, but one of the means where we feel we make the most impact is in our annual day of free dentistry, wherein we provide free fillings, extractions, or cleanings to members of the community who need it. The day is called Dentistry from the Heart, and it's not just our doctors providing voluntary services, but our entire team as we lend our skills to help those who need it most. This mentality of giving back is a part of our culture and one we're more than happy to nurture. It reminds us of how fortunate we are to do what we do, to work with the people we work with, and to be able to give, with our time, our knowledge, and our resources.

Dentistry from the Heart

Dentistry from the Heart began as a single event in the Tampa suburb of New Port Richey, Florida, in early 2001. The brainchild of Dr. Vincent Monticciolo, the intent of that first event was to provide relief to the many bay area residents that were in desperate need of dental care. The concept—which remains the same to this day—is to provide a free extraction, filling or cleaning to whoever needs it, no questions asked.

"Most patients opt for the extraction," said Michelle Sotil, director for Dentistry from the Heart. "Usually because they're dealing with some form of untreated dental disease or another condition that requires immediate attention."

The day of the first event, Dr. Monticciolo pulled up to his office to find a line around the block, with some having stood there since the night before in order to be first in line for the free services. The event was so successful that other practices throughout Florida began picking it up and from there, the event has spread to dental practices throughout the world.

As of 2018, there were more than three hundred Dentistry from the Heart events held in Canada each year, as well as in the United States, Ireland, New Zealand, Australia, and Puerto Rico.

"It's truly a wonderful charity, and each year it gets bigger," said Ms. Sotil.

While Dentistry from the Heart is a one-day event, participants in need of additional care are typically given information on nearby dental schools and free clinics for follow up treatment.[21]

The Impact of a Free Day of Dentistry

Steven was the sixteenth person waiting in line for a Dentistry from the Heart day. He was twenty-five years old and for the past five months, he'd been suffering from pain on the right side of his lower jaw. When we finally got him in a chair, the infection was so bad that extraction was really the only option.

Although no one is ever happy to lose a tooth, Steven was grateful for the service, stating that if it wasn't for the free day of dentistry, he wouldn't have been able to afford to have the tooth removed as he'd lost his job months ago and was having trouble finding work. In fact, a cousin of his went to the emergency room for a tooth infection a few months back, only to learn that the ER wasn't equipped to handle dental issues, which is the case with most emergency rooms across the country.

Low Income Adults and Poor Dental Health

According to a report by the American Dental Association's Health Policy Institute, of the low income adults surveyed:

- 35 percent are embarrassed about the condition of their mouth and teeth
- 42 percent have difficulty biting and chewing

---

21 Jody, "Dentistry From The Heart: From Day-of-Care Event to International Dental Nonprofit," Dentistry From The Heart, last modified August 10, 2017, http://dentistryfromtheheart.org/blog/director-of-dentistry-from-the-heart-michelle-sotil/

- 29 percent believe that the appearance of their mouth affects their ability to interview for a job
- 74 percent accept that they'll lose teeth with age, compared to 48 percent of high income adults
- Pain is the number one oral health problem suffered[22]

Unfortunately, this story isn't unusual. According to the American Dental Association, (ADA) "most hospitals don't have the facilities or staff to provide comprehensive dental care. So many patients receive only antibiotics or pain medication, but the underlying dental problem is not addressed. In too many cases, the patient returns to the emergency room with the same problem—or worse."[23]

Emergency room visits for dental pain have increased significantly over the years, with 2.1 million visits in 2010. Most of these were for non-traumatic dental conditions, and a 2015 ADA report estimates that up to 79 percent of dental-related ER visits could have been diverted to dental offices.[24] These statistics are very similar here in Canada.

---

22 "Oral Health and Well-Being in the United States," American Dental Association's Health Policy Institute, last modified 2015, http://www.ada.org/~/media/ADA/Science%20and%20Research/HPI/OralHealthWell-Being-StateFacts/US-Oral-Health-Well-Being.pdf?la=en

23 "From the Emergency Room to the Dental Chair," American Dental Association, http://www.ada.org/en/public-programs/action-for-dental-health/er-referral

24 Thomas Wall, Kamyar Nasseh, and Marko Vujicic, "Majority of Dental-Related Emergency Department Visits Lack Urgency and Can Be Diverted to Dental Offices," American Dental Association's Health Policy Institute, August 2014, http://www.ada.org/~/media/ADA/Science%20and%20Research/HPI/Files/HPIBrief_0814_1.ashx

Preventable Dental Emergencies

Dental ER visits doubled from 1.1 million in 2000 to 2.2 million in 2012

2000   2012

ER visits cost 3 times as much as dental visits

dental visit   ER visit

80% of dental-related ER visits are due to preventable conditions

Up to 1.05 million ER visits can be referred to dental clinics

Source: American Dental Association, ADA.org

What the ADA goes on to point out is that an increasing number of adults are forgoing regular dental care for a number of reasons, including the fact that dental benefits coverage has continued to decline for working-age adults.[25]

"The problem, while worse among lower income brackets, affects people across the economic spectrum," the ADA states, which is just one reason why programs such as Dentistry from the Heart are becoming increasingly important.[26]

---

25 Thomas Wall and Marko Vujicic, "Emergency Department Use for Dental Conditions Continues to Increase," American Dental Association's Health Policy Institute, April 2015, http://www.ada.org/~/media/ADA/Science%20and%20Research/HPI/Files/HPIBrief_0415_2.pdf?la=en

26 "From the Emergency Room to the Dental Chair," American Dental Association, http://www.ada.org/en/public-programs/action-for-dental-health/er-referral

How We Participate

In 2018, Dentistry from the Heart founder Dr. Monticciolo provided care to more than five hundred people at his New Port Richey clinic. At our practice, we strive to help as many people as we can during our free day of dentistry event, which is held in Spring. Additionally, we're committed to donating 10 percent of our revenue each year to a worthy cause.

For more information on when our next free day of dentistry event takes place, please visit our website www.VillanovaDental.com.

Chapter Seven

BEGIN WITH THE END IN MIND

Dental health is incredibly important at every age, and at every stage in your life, you risk dental health issues. As we age, the risk rises, which is why it's our job to remind you that the decisions you make about your dental health today are going to stay with you for the rest of your life. If you neglect your teeth now, chances are that you'll need more work later down the road and if you neglect those bigger repairs, then you might end up being one of those ten-percenters without any teeth whatsoever.

Coming back to the importance of good stewardship, not only is it beneficial to see your dentist regularly, but it's also important to know the kinds of dental conditions that you can expect with age as your teeth wear, and as any work you've had done begins to break down and your gums begin to recede.

For instance, I've been shocked to have people come in that undoubtedly need a crown on a tooth, and yet they accuse me or my staff of making up the fact that they need it. But if you think about how cavities are cared for—cleaning out the diseased area and bonding in a filling every five to twenty years, depending on conditions—then after two, three, or even four decay removals and filling replacements, inevitably there won't be much tooth left to fill and a crown will be necessary.

We don't want this or any procedure to be a surprise to you. Instead, it is our job to teach you about the natural progression of dental care and at what stages you may expect to take some extra preventative steps to keep your mouth healthy over the long term.

You can eliminate a lot of pain, discomfort, and frequent visits to the dentist by being proactive about your dental health. Our goal is to educate you so that you never feel that we're trying to "get" you to do something you don't want to do.

Check out the chart on page 69. There, you can jump to the most common dental conditions that are occurring at your age. I would suggest that you read it so you can have a good understanding behind any of the suggestions we make to you the next time you visit our offices. If you choose not to take preventative measures, that's your decision to make. However, know that if you choose to neglect your teeth for long periods of time, then you should budget to fix your teeth and take care of any related health conditions that may arise because of that neglect.

The best way to think about this is to begin with the end in mind. As you near the end of your life, what kind of teeth do you want to have? If you're like most people, then what you want is to have real teeth and a real smile. And you can have that - if you first understand that it is your responsibility to achieve it. As dentists, we're simply your partner and a provider of solutions to help you achieve your goals. It's on you to take the actions necessary to make those goals happen.

Part Two

Your Mouth at Every Age

Dental Expectations at Every Age

Childhood

Ages 0-6

Teaching proper toothbrushing

Treating common dental emergencies

- Knocked out tooth
- Cracked tooth
- Tongue or lip bite
- Toothaches
- Objects stuck in teeth

Fluoride treatment

Ages 7-9

First orthodontic visit

Establishing proper eating habits—avoiding sugary drinks and foods

Applying dental sealant (painted on child's 1st & 2nd molars as they emerge)

Pre-Teens and Teenagers

Reinforcing proper eating habits

Greater likelihood of cavities

Hormonal impact on oral health

Ages 20-39

Increased risk for gingivitis

Risk of TMJ pain due to:

- Tooth movement or other dental conditions
- Injury
- Craniofacial muscle spasms
- Rheumatic disease
- Other factors that cause the temporomandibular joint to shift

Stress impacts on oral health

- Tooth grinding
- Cracked teeth

Maintaining orthodontic adjustments (such as wearing a retainer after braces)

Ages 40-59

Increased risk of periodontal disease

Maintaining annual comprehensive periodontal evaluation

Old cavities may have to be crowned, or the tooth removed/replaced

Increased risk of obstructive sleep apnea

Maintaining preventative dental care

Ages 60+

Risk of cavities and tooth loss increases

Risk of gum recession

Risk of dry mouth

Reapplying fluoride varnish

Dental implants and dentures

Impact of osteoporosis on oral health

Watching out for signs of oral cancer

Dental care and dementia

Dental concerns may seem to come up completely out of the blue, but more often than not, they've been around for a while—we either just didn't notice them before or chose to ignore them until the irritation or pain become too much to bear. That's one of the biggest problems with dental issues—you could have a cavity and not even realize it until it becomes so deep that it hits the nerve. Or you may have gingivitis and ignore that tinge of blood when you're brushing or flossing until it becomes a full on case of periodontal disease.

This is what I sometimes call the "treadmill of dental life." Decisions regarding your dental health can come at you so quickly that you have to make decisions that you don't want to make—such as extraction or surgery—because of the condition you're in. However, if you're consciously taking preventative actions on the front end, then that treadmill slows down and you either don't have to make those decisions, or you have a lot more time to consider your options because you're aware of the condition long before it becomes a serious issue.

In this section of the book, we'll look at many of the dental concerns that can occur over a lifetime and what you can be doing now to prevent them. Or, if you haven't taken preventative measures for some time (such as brushing regularly and seeing your dentist at least once a year), this section should give you an idea of what conditions to expect at your current life stage.

For more information, or if you'd like to book an appointment, please call us at (613) 836-9084 or contact us by email at Info@VillanovaDental.com.

Chapter Eight

CHILDHOOD

Everyone has a childhood memory of what their first dental visit was like, which is why parents today are looking to make that experience better. They want their kids to look forward to seeing the dentist, which is why one of the first things we tell new parents is to bring their children in by the age of one.

That may seem a little young, but think of this way: when babies are born, their mouths are sterile. Within hours, however, they're colonized with organisms that will stay with them for the rest of their life. These bacteria, protozoa, viruses, and yeasts are mostly harmless, but once they settle in, they start building a habitat that's more welcoming to other, less-harmless organisms. Once a baby cuts those first teeth, the bacteria that's most likely linked to tooth decay—*streptococcus mutans*—is also likely to make an appearance.[27]

One of our biggest concerns when a baby's teeth first start to come in is that of Baby Bottle Tooth Decay, also known as "bottle rot." This condition typically affects the upper front teeth and is caused by prolonged exposure to sugar-containing drinks—including milk (milk contains 12 grams of naturally occurring sugar per cup, otherwise known as lactose). Prolonged exposure can occur when a child is put to bed with a bottle, or if they use a bottle as a pacifier, and that sugar is the best way to activate the rapid growth of *streptococcus mutans*.

When sugar is present, *S. Mutans* feeds on it, releasing acids that can eventually eat away at tooth enamel, making room for plaque to grab ahold, which bacteria latch onto and from there, begin forming new holes. The more sugar that's added, the more this condition spreads until the mouth's natural cleanser—saliva—can no longer wash it away.

Even though a child will eventually lose his or her baby teeth, these first teeth play a very important role in life. They are needed for developing clear speech, chewing, and will also help the adult teeth come in correctly.

---

27   Jane E. Stevens, "Oral Ecology," MIT Technolgy Review, last modified January 1, 1997, https://www.technologyreview.com/s/400012/oral-ecology/

Toothbrushing and Dental Health Care for Ages 0–6

Infants

- For babies whose teeth have not emerged yet, use a clean, damp pad or washcloth to wipe your child's gums after each feeding.

- Only place formula, milk, or breast milk in bottles. Do not fill them with juice, sugar water, or soft drinks.

- Do not put an infant to sleep with a bottle. Bottles should be finished before nap time and bedtime.

- If an infant uses a pacifier, only give them a clean one—do not dip it in honey or other sugar-containing liquids.

1–3 years old

- When your child's teeth come in, use a child-size toothbrush and no more than a pinch (about the size of a grain of rice) of children's toothpaste to brush their teeth until three years of age.

- Encourage drinking from a cup

- Encourage healthy eating habits

3–7 years old

- Brush your child's teeth with a child's toothbrush and a pea-sized amount of children's toothpaste.

- If your child wishes to brush his or her own teeth, make sure to supervise the process to ensure that all of the teeth are brushed and all of the toothpaste is spit out instead of swallowed. Supervision should occur until the child is between the ages of six and seven.[28]

Dealing with Common Dental Emergencies

As many times as you've warned your child not to climb on top of the monkey bars, or open containers with his teeth, or ride his bike too fast (I could go on, but if you're a parent, you know what I mean), dental emergencies still occur. Here are a few ways to deal with them when they come up:

- **Knocked-out tooth**: try to put the tooth back in its socket without touching the root. If you can't, then either place the tooth in your child's cheek next to the gum, or if you're worried about the child swallowing the tooth, place it in a glass of milk. Then call your dentist immediately.

- **Cracked tooth**: rinse the mouth with warm water to clean it out and give the child a cold compress to place against the side of the mouth to keep any swelling down. Then call your dentist immediately.

- **Tongue or lip bite**: rinse the mouth with warm water and apply a cool or cold compress to the affected area.

- **Toothaches**: rinse the mouth with warm water and gently use dental floss to remove any food caught between teeth, as this can be exacerbating the pain. Call your dentist as soon as it is convenient.

- **Objects stuck in the teeth**: try to use floss to gently remove it, but if that does not work, call the dentist. Do not try to

---

28   "Baby Bottle Tooth Decay," Mouth Healthy, American Dental Association, http://www.mouthhealthy.org/en/az-topics/b/baby-bottle-tooth-decay

use a sharp, solid instrument to remove the object as it may cause further damage.

"Colorado Brown Stain" and the Introduction of Fluoride

You've probably heard me or other dentists talking about the importance of using toothpaste containing fluoride at every age, including those first toothbrushing years. There are a lot of reasons behind this, first and foremost that, while fluoride is added to tap water, very few people drink tap water anymore, opting instead for bottled water or filtered water (note, however, that "activated carbon" filters do not remove fluoride. Only processes such as reverse osmosis and deionization can remove the mineral).

Secondly, bottled water can be incredibly acidic. A study published in the Journal of Dental Hygiene found that, of the fourteen commercial bottled water brands tested, ten were acidic, with a pH of less than 7.

"Dental professionals continually educate patients on the dangers of consuming acidic food and drink due to their potential to contribute to dental erosion and tooth decay," the study noted, "However, water is not typically categorized as acidic." In investigating the pH values as reported on each of the bottled water manufacturers' websites, the researchers also found that the actual values were lower (more acidic) than those reported.

So why is fluoride added to water?

The discovery of fluoride and its dental benefits ironically began with the problems that fluoride was causing. In 1901, a young dentist named Frederick McKay arrived in Colorado Springs, Colorado, with the intention of opening a dental practice. What he found when he arrived was astonishing—the residents of the town had dark brown stains on their teeth, some so significant that "sometimes entire teeth were splotched the color of chocolate candy." Eventually, the condition became known as Colorado Brown Stain.

Apart from the colouration, however, the staining didn't seem to be causing any harm, and in fact, after years of research, McKay found that these mottled teeth were very resistant to cavity formation. Additionally, he found that city residents whose permanent teeth came in and calcified before the stains set in did not develop the stains later, so the staining had to occur while the teeth were developing.

It was later discovered that incredibly high levels of fluoride in the water were causing the brown stain—a condition that became known as "fluorosis." But lower levels of fluoride didn't stain and actually appeared to be beneficial. Later on, studies confirmed that fluoride ions easily absorb into the surface of teeth where demineralization has occurred, and bond with the enamel. The bonded fluoride then attracts other minerals, such as calcium, to the damaged area, thereby strengthening the tooth overall.

The next question to answer, then, was how the benefits of fluoride could be used without triggering the ugly staining caused by fluorosis. Decades after the cause of fluorosis was discovered, Dr. H. Trendley Dean, head of the Dental Hygiene Unit at the National Health Institute, began to study exactly how much fluoride needed to be in water before fluorosis occurred, and whether or not physically and cosmetically safe levels of fluoride in water would help fight tooth decay.

In 1945, Dean worked out a deal with Grand Rapids, Michigan, to safely fluoridate the town's drinking water over a fifteen-year period. After eleven years, Dean was able to confirm that children born in Grand Rapids after the fluoride was introduced were 60 percent less likely to develop cavities.

Today, fluoridation projects benefit millions of Canadians and fluoride can be found in just about every toothpaste brand on the market.

Ages 7–9: First Orthodontic Visit

The best time for a child's first orthodontic visit is between the ages of seven and nine. This may seem like an odd time since most children still have quite a few of their baby teeth at this age, but this is actually the perfect age to have a preliminary screening done to ensure that there are no issues developing, such as crossbites, over-, or under-bites.

If there is an issue, this age is also the ideal time to start Phase One Treatment, which focuses less on the teeth and more on changing jaw growth. The younger a child is, the easier it is to guide the jaw into a stable, ideal bite. Imagine how much more growth a seven year old has ahead of him or her, rather than a twelve or thirteen-year-old—when potential issues are caught during this window of opportunity, we can get a jump on corrections and reduce the amount of time that child will need to spend in braces later on.

Ages 6–12: Dental Sealant

Dental sealants are thin coatings painted on a child's first and second molars (which emerge around the ages of six and age twelve, respectively) that fill in the deep grooves of the tooth to prevent cavities. According to the Center for Disease Control (CDC), "once applied, sealants protect against 80 percent of cavities for two years and continue to protect against 50 percent of cavities for up to four years." This is particularly important as the permanent back teeth are where nine out of every ten cavities occur.

---

*Top Three Tooth-Rotting Beverages**

Sports Drinks

Sweetened Iced Tea Drinks

Energy Drinks

People always say "Don't drink soda because of the sugar" but the truth of the matter is that a sugar-free energy drink is worse for your teeth than a classic cola, because it's more acidic. It's that combination of sugar and acid that does the most damage, but acid is ultimately worse on your teeth than sugar.

Chapter Nine

PRE-TEENS AND TEENAGERS

The pre-teen years are when you really reinforce the importance of brushing teeth twice a day on their own. At this point, your child should have already had their first orthodontist visit and may or may not be undergoing treatment to prevent a bite condition. Of all the things you can do for your child's dental health at this age, having sealant applied is one of the most important, if only for the long-term impact that this pretty simple process can have.

Eating for a Healthy Mouth

When it comes to maintaining overall mouth health, diet and nutrition are just as important as good brushing habits. Diet (the food we eat) and nutrition (the nutrients in the food) both impact the health of our mouth differently. Diet has a local effect, impacting the integrity of our teeth, saliva, and the mouth's pH balance, while nutrition has more of a systemic effect, impacting the integrity of the jaw bone, teeth, and supporting structure of the teeth. That is, changing your diet will more directly affect your mouth health while changes in nutrition will also have an impact, but it will happen over a longer period of time and affect the greater structure of the mouth.

Where we often run into trouble is the overconsumption of what's called "fermentable carbohydrates," which are those added and naturally occurring sugars in food. The difference between fermentable carbohydrates and other carbohydrates is that the fermentable kind breaks down in the mouth instead of later on in the digestive tract, sticking around to feed bacteria and launch the decay process.

Fermentable carbohydrates come in obvious and not-so-obvious forms. There are those foods that definitely contain sugar, such as candies, cakes, cookies, sodas, and chocolates. And then there are the less-obvious: bread, breakfast cereal, bananas, crackers, potato chips, pretzels and even dried fruit.

Additionally, the "stickier" these fermentable carbs are, the worse they are for your mouth, as they latch on to the nooks and crannies of the tooth and feed the bacteria that produces the acid that eats away at tooth enamel. "Sticky" doesn't just mean gooey and gummy in the way raisins and licorice are sticky—it can also mean "gets stuck easily" in the way potato chip crumbs can become wedged between your teeth and stick around long after you've finished eating them.

What are the best foods to eat for a wholesome diet, good nutrition, and an overall healthy mouth? The dietary guidelines in the Canada Food Guide is a great place to start:

A healthy eating pattern **includes**:

- A variety of dark green, red, and orange vegetables
- Legumes (peas and beans)
- Grains, at least half of which are whole (brown rice, oatmeal, whole wheat bread)
- Fresh, whole fruits
- Low-fat or fat-free dairy, including milk, cheese, yogurt
- Protein foods, including seafood, poultry, eggs, lean meat, nuts, seeds, and soy products

A healthy eating pattern **limits** saturated fats, trans fats, added sugars and sodium, and includes consuming:

- Less than 10 percent of daily calories from added sugars
- Less than 10 percent of daily calories from saturated fats
- Less than 2,300 mg of sodium per day

If alcohol is consumed by adults of legal drinking age, it should be limited to one drink per day for women, and two drinks per day for men.

Every diet should begin with a strong base of grains as well as a daily intake of:

- 2 1/2 cups of vegetables
- 2 cups of fresh fruit
- 3 cups of calcium-containing milk, yogurt, and/or cheese
- Proteins (meats, beans, eggs, nuts)

And when it comes to snacking, try to choose non-sticky, non-fermentable carbohydrates. For example:

Best choice:

- Cheese
- Protein (meats, beans, eggs, nuts)
- Milk products (no sugar added)
- Water

Okay choice:

- Whole fruits such as apples and pears (these contain natural sugars, but have enough water in them that the sugar is diluted and saliva can more easily wash them out of the mouth)
- Vegetables (while vegetables contain carbs, they don't have enough to be dangerous)
- Unsweetened carbonated waters (these often contain a small amount of sodium)

Worst choice:

- Candy
- Cookies
- Crackers

- Bread

- Muffins

- Potato chips

- Pretzels

- Dried fruit

- Bananas

- French fries

- Cakes

- Soft drinks and other drinks containing sugar, including fruit juices

Ages 13–19: Treating Cavities

When lunch consists of a trip to the convenience store for a soda and a candy bar, cavities are eventually going to be an issue. A lot of teenage boys are full on into not taking care of themselves, and while girls tend to do a better job of taking care of themselves and their dental health, cavities can still become an issue—particularly if you have a family history of dental conditions.

Even though kids should already be seeing their dentist twice a year, this age range is when a bi-yearly checkup becomes incredibly important. Cavities need to be caught early and treated before they lead to further tooth decay.

When it comes to fillings, preference in Canada has more or less shifted away from silver amalgam and toward composite fillings, though there are a number of filling options available, and the procedure itself is pretty simple.

Types of Fillings

Depending on your preferences, the extent of tooth decay, and whether or not you have any allergies to certain materials such as metals, there are a number of options for filling materials, including:

- **Gold**: While expensive, gum tissues actually tolerate gold incredibly well and the fillings can last in excess of twenty years. However, apart from the cost, gold fillings also take longer as they often have to be made to order by a third-party lab before they can be cemented into place. This can require multiple visits before the procedure is complete.

- **Silver (amalgam)**: Also a material that's pretty resistant to wear, silver fillings also tolerate the heat and moisture of the mouth well, are relatively inexpensive, and last an average of fifteen years. However, since they're dark in color, they're more noticeable. Compositionally, most silver fillings are composed of mercury, silver, tin, copper, and other trace metals. Over time, due to shrinkage and expansion, they can cause cracks to form in teeth.

- **Composite**: This is increasingly the most used filling type as the color is much closer to the natural color of the tooth. They have an average lifespan of three to ten years depending on care, and common liquids such as coffee and tea can cause them to stain. "Composite" is short for "composite resins," which is usually a combination of specialized plastics and a filler such as silica.

- **Porcelain**: Like gold, porcelain inlays typically need to be custom created by a lab and then bonded to the tooth. These fillings can be matched to the exact color of the tooth and can last between fifteen and thirty years. By nature, porcelain is also resistant to staining.

Basic Filling Procedure

1. The process of cleaning and filling a cavity begins with local anesthesia, which is used to numb the area around the tooth so that you don't feel pain during the process.

2. Then we clean out the decay using a small drill and shape the space so the filling will fit in tightly. If we're doing a bonded filling, we'll also etch the tooth with an acid gel before placing the filling.

3. Finally, we'll place the filling and polish the tooth to ensure that the filling is smooth and comfortable.

How Puberty (Hormones) Can Affect Your Teeth

Along with all the other changes your body goes through during puberty, one of the more overlooked ones is the change that happens with your gums.

Between the ages of eleven and thirteen, when puberty is most likely to occur, gum tissue becomes more responsive to the accumulation of dental plaque and may bleed and become inflamed more frequently. When these symptoms become more prevalent, the condition is generally referred to as chronic marginal gingivitis, or puberty gingivitis, and it's generally believed to be caused by the increased hormone levels that occur with puberty*.

Both males and females are susceptible to the condition, and its onset is believed to be predictive of the formation of more significant periodontal diseases later in life.

This is just another reason why good dental health is incredibly important in the pre-teen and teenage years, as proper oral hygiene today can be the difference between healthy teeth and gums for a lifetime.

*Of note, the hormonal changes that can occur with pregnancy and menopause have also been associated with an increased risk of gingivitis and periodontal disease.

Chapter Ten

AGES 20–39

The college years are another span of life where cavities are more likely to appear. The typical college diet doesn't help, with late-night study snacks coming into play more often and the general neglect of leafy green vegetables in one's diet. College is also when gum disease starts to pop up, starting out with the light bleeding of the gums during brushing, which is caused by gingivitis. If left untreated, those irritated, inflamed gums can quickly evolve into full on periodontal disease.

The good news is that gingivitis is pretty reversible during this age range. If you can get back into regular dental visits, regular cleanings, and brushing your teeth at least twice a day, the inflammation can go away without any permanent damage. If, however, the gingivitis goes for too long untreated, then not only will your teeth need to be cleaned, but your gums, as well, which is a much bigger deal. Think of it as similar to the condition that your car would be in if you didn't wash it for five or six years. You can't just drive that kind of buildup through the car wash and expect it all to come off—you have to get some serious detail work done.

What are the signs of gingivitis?

That little bit of blood in your toothpaste every time you spit? That's not supposed to be there. Gingivitis is the swelling and irritation of the gingiva, which is the part of your gum at the base of your teeth, and if it's not taken care of quickly it can lead to tooth loss, periodontitis, and other serious gum diseases.

Apart from a bit of blood when you brush, other signs and symptoms of gingivitis include:

- Puffy, swollen gums

- Dark red gums

- Tender gums

- Bad breath

- Receding gumline[29]

Gingivitis begins most often with poor dental health. When the biofilm on teeth isn't brushed away regularly, it can build up to form plaque, and that plaque is what causes irritation. Then, as the plaque builds, it turns into calculus—otherwise known as tartar—which is much more difficult to remove than plaque and is a breeding ground for bacteria. Only a professional dental cleaning can remove calculus. If that calculus isn't addressed, it will begin to irritate the gingiva, causing irritation, which then allows the gums to bleed more easily.

29   "Gingivitis," Mayo Clinic, https://www.mayoclinic.org/diseases-conditions/ gingivitis/symptoms-causes/syc-20354453

This bleeding then opens the door to more bacteria getting directly into the gums and the bloodstream, leading to tooth loss, periodontitis and the risk of those diseases we mentioned earlier.

What increases the risk of gingivitis?

Poor brushing habits are the most common risk factor for gingivitis, but other conditions can contribute to the risk, including:

- Dry mouth

- Poor nutrition

- Dental restorations that don't fit well

- Crooked teeth that aren't cleaned well

- Conditions that cause a decrease in immunity such as HIV/AIDS, leukemia, or cancer treatment

- Smoking or chewing tobacco

- Old age

- Hormonal changes

- Genetics

- Viral and fungal infections

Headaches or TMJ Pain?

Of all of the hinging points in your body, the temporomandibular joint (TMJ, commonly called the "jaw joint") works harder than any other. Also, due to the combination of sliding motions and hinging, the TMJ is also the most complicated joint in the body. The jaw joint is where all of the major movements of your skull are centered and it is constantly moving, whether you're aware of it or not. On a conscious level, its active when we chew, speak, or yawn, and on a subconscious level its constantly making micro movements such as clenching, grinding, shifting, and repeatedly opening and closing.

Due to its connection to the trigeminal nerve—the largest of the twelve cranial nerves which run throughout the upper and lower jaws and into the teeth, eyes, and even the tongue—the smallest misalignment can have a significant impact on the rest of the system.

There are numerous conditions that may lead to TMJ pain, many of which become more prevalent as we age. These include:

- **Tooth movement or dental conditions** – tooth movement as we age, the wearing down of teeth, and tooth replacement, as well as dental procedures that change how our teeth interact, can affect the TMJ

- **Injury** – trauma to the jaw joint, head, or neck can have long-term effects that may not be felt until months or possibly years after the initial injury occurred

- **Craniofacial muscle spasms** – caused by injury or medications

- **Rheumatic disease** – this condition, which refers to a larger group of conditions that cause inflammation, pain, and stiffness of the joints, such as arthritis, can affect the TMJ as a secondary condition.

Common signs of TMJ issues:

- Facial aches and pains
- Frequent headaches
- Tooth wear

- Numerous dental problems (broken teeth, crowns or history of several root canals)
- Aches and pains around the ear
- Tender or painful jaw
- Discomfort or difficulty chewing
- Popping, clicking or grinding noise in jaw joints
- Difficulty opening and closing mouth due to locking of jaw joint

A significant sports injury in your teenage years or early twenties, or a car accident that seemed to only result in a case of whiplash, may evolve into issues with the TMJ later in life as the damaged jaw joint deteriorates under the tension of the unbalanced system.

What causes TMJ Pain?

Any time your bite changes, it affects your TMJ, and anytime your TMJ shifts, it can put mechanical stress on your teeth. Think of it like a finely tuned engine—if anything becomes misaligned, however slight, it will put stress on the system. As the stress increases over time, the misalignment becomes worse until the whole system becomes noticeably and painfully out of alignment.

Patterns of dental problems on the back teeth in particular can be a sign of undiagnosed TMJ issues. These problems can include root canals, missing back teeth, cracked teeth, broken porcelain fillings, etc, any of which can indicate that the system is under more stress than it should be. Additionally, teeth that are under additional stress from excessive bite force are also more likely to suffer periodontal problems.

One of the biggest problems with TMJ issues is how long they take to manifest. If headaches due to an injury that affected the TMJ don't appear until years after the incident, then it's not likely that the person suffering from them is going to make that connection.

Good dentists should be on the lookout for these types of conditions. If the alignment of the patient's jaw seems off, even if it's just slight, and we suspect a TMJ issue, then the first thing we'll do is test the diagnosis. This typically involves the patient being fitted with a type of appliance called an orthotic, which sets the jaw joint back into an ideal bite when worn.

An orthotic does more than just protect the teeth from grinding together at night. Instead, it is custom designed to hold the jaw in just the right position so that the teeth are aligned, relieving the muscle stress being placed on the TMJ by the misalignment.

After a few months of relief and time to stabilize, we move into more permanent treatment options to make the correction and relief permanent and last a lifetime.

Home Care for TMJ Issues

If you suspect that you have TMJ issues, there are some steps you can take at home to relieve the discomfort:

- Ice packs applied to the side of the face, particularly just in front of the ear where the TMJ is located
- Make conscious efforts to keep your face relaxed with lips together and teeth apart
- Eat softer foods
- Take small bites and chew with both sides of the mouth
- Don't rest your chin in your hand

- Don't bite hard objects, such as pencils, fingernails, cuticles, etc.

- Don't hold phones between the neck and shoulder

- Avoid excessive or extensive movements of the jaw, such as big yawns or chewing gum.

- Practice stress-relieving techniques

- Do gentle jaw stretches or jaw massages. One approach is to place your thumb or fingertip in the small "notch" located about one inch in front of your ears and on the underside of the cheekbone. Gently pressing inward and upward in this spot and rubbing in soft circular motions may provide some relief.

If the TMJ pain continues, there are other options for treatment, though each should only be considered after assessing all of the pros, cons, and risks with your doctor:

- **Pain medication:** muscle relaxers, pain killers and other medications as prescribed may help with the temporary relief of TMJ pain.

- **Dental adjustments:** this involves making changes to the teeth to bring the bite back into balance.

- **Botox**: Since Botox works by blocking the nerve signals to the muscles, it may provide temporary relief to sore jaw muscles when used in small doses, although this method is not approved by the FDA for use with TMJ issues.

- **Surgery**: While surgery is an option, it should be avoided where possible as there are no long-term clinical trials showing the effectiveness of surgical procedures helping with TMJ disorders, and the treatment is often irreversible.

- **Implants**: Artificial implants to replace jaw joints are also an option, but should also be taken under the same strict considerations as surgery.

For more information on discussions around TMJ treatments, give us a call at (613) 836-9084 or email us at info@VillanovaDental.com.

Stressed Out? Your Teeth are Probably Feeling the Pressure

"I sheared off my front tooth," actor Demi Moore explained to *Tonight Show* host Jimmy Fallon during a show back in June 2017. "I'd love to say it was skateboarding or something really kind of cool, but I think it's something that's important to share because I think it's literally, probably after heart disease, one of the biggest killers in America, which is stress."[30]

While stress doesn't immediately cause your teeth to fracture, loosen, or fall out, it can cause this kind of damage over time, with stress increasingly becoming more prevalent in younger generations.[31] Under high stress, people may forget to brush or floss, and may not have the time or even think to visit the dentist. The same conditions can also lead to increased cortisol levels in the body, and while cortisol in the short term has an anti-inflammatory effect, extended or exaggerated stress response can lead to cortisol dysfunction, which can result in widespread inflammation and pain.

---

30 Bruce Lee, "Demi Moore Lost Two Teeth To Stress, Here's How It Can Happen," Forbes, last modified June 15, 2017, https://www.forbes.com/sites/brucelee/2017/06/15/demi-moore-lost-two-teeth-to-stress-heres-how-it-can-happen/

31 "2015 Stress in America," American Psychological Association, http://www.apa.org/news/press/releases/stress/2015/snapshot.aspx

Stress can also exacerbate bruxism, which is the medical term for teeth grinding. If you apply enough force to your teeth, over a long enough period of time, you can do significant damage. On average, a human can bite down with two hundred pounds of force per square inch, which is actually pretty powerful, and when you apply that kind force regularly on just about anything, it's going to cause some damage.

To understand how that kind of pressure affects the mouth, consider how this part of the body is composed. The tissues surrounding the teeth, for instance, are basically tight strands similar to guitar strings, holding everything together. But when you put excessive pressure on guitar strings, what happens? They pop, which is basically what is happening to the tissues around your teeth when you clench and grind. This is why the gums start to recede around teeth affected by bruxism, as the forces cause those tissues to break. If those forces continue, they go on to wear away the enamel, exposing the dentin and creating access points for bacteria to get directly into the blood stream.

Bruxism can occur consciously or subconsciously, while you're awake or asleep, and may not seem to be a concern for months or even years after it first starts to occur.

Signs of bruxism include:

- Dull headaches (especially in the morning)

- Sore jaw muscles

- Pain radiating from the ear

- Teeth sensitivity

- Chipped, cracked teeth

- Loose teeth

- Damage on the inside of the cheek from chewing or biting

- Indentations in the tongue

While bruxism is common in younger children, the condition is usually temporary and more likely due to allergies, teething, or misaligned baby teeth as opposed to stress. Most children outgrow teeth grinding by their teens.

If bruxism continues, or if you suffer from it as an adult, then the long-term pressure and grinding of the teeth can lead to chipping, cracks, and loose teeth that may eventually fall out, as well as the wearing down of the enamel. In severe cases, the enamel can become so worn that the underlying layer of dentin is exposed. This not only causes sensitivity, but the dentin, which is nine times softer than enamel, is much more susceptible to decay.

In rare cases, long-term bruxing can lead to the enlargement of facial muscles, which can block the salivary glands, leading to swelling, pain, inflammation, and dry mouth. And dry mouth alone is a major trigger for cavity formation as the lack of saliva means that the mouth doesn't have its natural means of regular cleansing available to it.

While stress can certainly result in bruxism, teeth grinding can also be related to sleep issues or any of those childhood conditions listed earlier, such as a misaligned bite or allergies. Most commonly, grinding is a symptom of TMD (a bad bite). In milder cases, bruxism may not necessarily need treatment. But if the problem persists to the point of discomfort, jaw pain, and damage to the teeth, then one or multiple forms of treatment may be recommended.

Treating Teeth Grinding (Bruxism)

Dental treatment

Although dental treatment may help to relieve the effect of bruxism, it won't necessarily treat the cause. Some options include:

- **Mouth guards and occlusal splints**: mouth guards can protect your teeth from grinding directly against each other while you sleep, and occlusal splints can be custom built to keep your teeth in an ideal bite position, as well as prevent direct contact of teeth during sleep.

- **Dental correction**: if the degree of bruxism has lead to teeth becoming so sensitive that you can no longer drink hot or cold liquids or chew properly, then the teeth may need to be reshaped and restored in order to repair the damage. This ideally would be done in a harmonious, physiologic relationship.

Behavior modification

If stress is a likely cause of bruxism, behavioral medication and management may help:

- **Stress management**: learning strategies that promote relaxation such as meditation, may help to reduce anxiety, which may have a positive impact on bruxism.

- **Behavior modification**: if you're aware of bruxism and how it's manifesting in your jaw habits, then you may be able to change that behavior by practicing proper jaw positioning, as demonstrated by your dentist.

- **Biofeedback**: through the use of electrical sensors, you can view information on how your body is reacting to subtle changes, which may help in reducing those actions that result in bruxing. For instance, learning how to consciously control your breathing and heart rate can be a helpful calming technique, and learning how to effectively relax the mouth and jaw muscles may reduce the effects of bruxism, or help to eliminate it altogether if it's main source is stress and muscle tension.

- **Lifestyle modifications**: some at-home methods for reducing the factors that contribute to bruxism can include:

  - Taking relaxing baths, listening to soothing music or exercising

  - Avoiding stimulating substances such as alcohol or coffee in the evening

  - Getting a good night's sleep

  - Asking your sleep partner to let you know if they hear you making any grinding noises, or if your jaw is clicking at night, so you can inform your dentist or doctor

  - Schedule regular dental exams to spot signs of bruxism early

By addressing teeth grinding earlier in life, you're more likely to avoid its longer-term impacts, and more likely to make it into your later years with most, if not all, of your natural teeth.

Retaining that Smile

If you had braces as a teenager, it's likely that your dentist played an important part in keeping your teeth clean between orthodontic visits, and reporting any concerns, breaks or other conditions to your orthodontist. However, in my office, I am able to oversee both duties.

After the braces come off, the relationship between me and my patients continue, as the patients are monitored to ensure that the braces did what they were intended to do—and a big part of that has to do with whether or not the patient is good about wearing a retainer.

It's a tough ask for a teenager who just got out of braces to continue wearing another appliance, but the first year after braces is vital for ensuring that the teeth are secure in their new locations. This is why I recommend that you wear your retainer up to twenty-two hours every day for the first three to six months, then every night at least for the following six months. Most kids are pretty good about that extra year—its the time afterward that presents the most challenge.

If you wore braces as a kid, you should still be wearing your retainer at least three nights a week and ideally every night for the rest of your life.

This is because, even with all of that time in braces, your teeth are going to shift. It may take a couple decades, but your teeth will gradually shift forward and inward with age—unless you have gingivitis or periodontal disease, in which case your teeth will shift much sooner than that.

If, by chance, you have been wearing your retainer regularly since your teenage years, then the other caveat of maintaining that healthy straight smile is getting your retainer replaced as needed; every two to ten years, depending on how rough you are on them. This isn't just because the retainer can wear out, however—it's also because of the inevitable tooth drift that occurs as you get older. Even with retention, teeth are going to shift slightly and the retainer will need to be adjusted in order to keep those teeth in proper alignment.

Over the course of a lifetime, you may go through several retainers, but wearing a retainer at night a few nights out of the week is a small price to pay for the long-term benefit of keeping your teeth straight and healthy.

Chapter Eleven

AGES 40–59

For most of us, that feeling of invincibility that we've had our whole lives is likely starting to wear off in this stage—and our systems are starting to wind down a little along with it.

On the brighter side, this is the stage of life where a lot of us start taking better care of our bodies. Before this age, parents in particular were putting their children's health ahead of their own, making sure the kids went to the doctor and dentist regularly while neglecting their own health. Once the kids start to grow up, however— and in some cases move out of the house—moms and dads start to reinvest in making themselves look and feel better, working on getting their looks as close to—or better than—they were in their pre-kid days. This likely means more working out and more time at the dentist, looking into what can not only be done health-wise but also cosmetically.

Unfortunately, this is also the age when people who were neglecting the signs and symptoms of gingivitis are now likely suffering from full-on periodontal disease.

What is Periodontal Disease (Periodontitis)?

Periodontal disease occurs when gingivitis isn't treated, and the gums pull away from the teeth, forming spaces that then become infected. In fact, the word "periodontitis" means "inflammation around the tooth." As the infection grows, the toxins and the immune system begin to break down the bone and tissues holding the infected teeth in place, eventually leading to tooth loss.

The signs and symptoms of periodontal disease are the same as gingivitis—as are the risk factors. Treatment, too, follows the same path, beginning with a complete deep cleaning that involves scraping the tartar from above and below the gum line, and removing rough spots on the tooth root where germs gather. In some cases, a laser may be used to remove all of the offending buildup.

Antibiotic and antimicrobial medications may also be recommended after a deep cleaning, but if the damage is too extensive, surgery is most likely the next step.

Surgical Treatments for Periodontal Disease

There are two main types of surgical procedures for periodontal disease. Depending on the extent of the damage, your dentist may recommend:

Flap Surgery

This procedure involves lifting back the gums to remove extensive tartar deposits, followed by suturing the gums back into place so that everything fits tightly. Once healed, the gums should fit snug around the tooth and the teeth may appear longer as a result.

Bone & Tissue Grafts

Sometimes flap surgery isn't enough, however, particularly when the disease has eaten away at the gum tissue and even the bone underneath. Bone grafting involves placing a piece of natural or synthetic bone in the area of bone loss in order to stimulate growth. In some cases, guided tissue regeneration may also be used, which involves placing a piece of mesh between the gum and bone that blocks the gum tissue from growing where the bone should be, giving the bone and connective tissue time to grow. A graft of soft tissue may also be used for gum loss, with synthetic material or tissue from another part of the mouth being used to cover exposed tooth roots.

The success of either procedure is entirely dependent on the patient, his or her risk factors and how well mouth health is maintained at home going forward.[32]

Believe it or not, one out of every two Americans over the age of thirty have some stage of periodontitis, which the more advanced form of periodontal disease. And in adults over the age of sixty-five, the prevalence is a little over 70 percent of all Americans.[33] These statistics are very similar to those in Canada.

Interestingly enough, according to study conducted in part by the Centers for Disease Control (CDC), men are more likely than women to have periodontal disease (56.4 percent vs. 38.4 percent in women), and those at the highest risk include current smokers (64.2

---

32   "Periodontal (Gum) Disease: Causes, Symptoms, and Treatments," National Institute of Dental and Craniofacial Research, last modified September 2013, https://www.nidcr.nih.gov/OralHealth/Topics/GumDiseases/PeriodontalGumDisease.htm

33   "CDC: Half of American Adults Have Periodontal Disease," American Academy of Periodontology, https://www.perio.org/consumer/cdc-study.htm

percent), those with less than a high school education (66.9 percent) and those living below the federal poverty level (65.4 percent).

"Periodontal disease is associated with age," stated Paul Eke, MPH, PhD, lead author of the study and CDC epidemiologist, "and as Americans live longer and retain more of their natural teeth, periodontal disease may take on more prominence in the oral health of the U.S. Adult population. Maintaining good periodontal health is important to the overall health and well-being of our aging population."

With these findings, co-author Robert Genco, DDS, PhD, believes that periodontal disease should be elevated to the level of Public Health Concern. "We now know that periodontal disease is one of the most prevalent, non-communicable chronic diseases in our population, similar to cardiovascular disease and diabetes," Genco stated.[34]

Have You Had Your Annual Comprehensive Periodontal Evaluation?

According to the American Academy of Periodontology, every dental patient should have a comprehensive periodontal evaluation conducted on annual basis to gauge periodontal health, diagnose existing disease, assess risk for disease, and determine any needed treatment. This service can be conducted during a regular dental visit by the general dentist, or by a dental hygienist or periodontist.

---

34 P.I. Eke et al., "Prevalence of Periodontitis in Adults in the United States: 2009 and 2010," *Journal of Dental Research* 91, no. 10 (August 2012), https://doi.org/10.1177/0022034512457373

Crowning Moment

If you've had cavities since you were a kid, then crowns are very likely in your near future. Between the ages of forty and sixty is when most fillings have run their effective course. If you've been keeping up with your dental visits, then a cavity that you had filled in your pre-teens or teens was likely redone in your twenties or early thirties. Depending on the original size of the cavity, the redo of that filling will likely take away significantly more of the surrounding structure. Then, when the cavity needs to be replaced again in, say, ten to fifteen years, then there's a good chance that there won't be enough tooth structure left for a filling, and a crown will need to be placed instead.

The fact of the matter is that if you have a cavity, you're going to end up with a crown. It might be sooner, if the cavity is bigger or if you are particularly rough on your teeth, or it might be later—but it's almost always necessary.

Snoring Problem or Obstructive Sleep Apnea?

While obstructive sleep apnea can occur at any age, the risk factor increases with age and the condition is more prevalent in men over the age of forty. While this may not seem like a condition that you would immediately think to bring up with your dentist, we're actually in one of the best positions to help with this disorder as treatment often involves adjusting the jaw in order to open up the airway and increase airflow.

Obstructive sleep apnea, or OSA, is a medical condition in which the sufferer stops breathing for seconds up to minutes at a time while sleeping. These pauses in breathing, called "apneas," can occur thirty or more times in an hour, and breathing often starts again with a loud choking sound or snort. This disruption may not entirely wake the person up, but it will move them from a deep sleep to a light slight sleep, which greatly reduces the overall quality of their sleep and leads to excessive daytime sleepiness.

Even though OSA is a common condition, it often goes undiagnosed as those who suffer from it don't realize it's occurring unless someone tells them. And if a sleep partner does notice, they often write it off as loud snoring instead of something more. If you're concerned that someone is suffering from OSA, the best way to tell is by listening for that pause in breathing between snores. Snoring is usually only a split-second closure of the upper airway that doesn't interrupt the sleeper, while OSA sufferers will noticeably stop breathing before starting again.

Along with that audible pause, other signs and symptoms of the condition include:

- lower jaw is too small or is set too far back

- excessive sleepiness

- fatigue

- memory impairment

- mood disturbance

- decreased libido

- social withdrawal

- cardiovascular disease

- presence of hypertension

- BMI of 30 or higher

- neck circumference of 17 inches or larger

- observed choking or gasping during sleep

- inattention and changes in energy levels during the day

- enlarged tonsils and/or adenoids

There is also evidence that people who suffer from bruxism—teeth grinding—may also have some degree of OSA as that jaw movement may be related to the subconscious effort to keep the airway open during sleep, moving the jaw around or clenching the it in order to activate the throat and neck muscles and keep the airway open.

Diagnosing Obstructive Sleep Apnea

The method for determining if someone is suffering from sleep apnea is typically two parts: a basic sleep screening followed by a sleep study conducted with a polysomnograph, or PSG.

The sleep screening can be conducted at the dentist office and usually involves a series of questions or situations to determine someone's daytime sleepiness scale. Two of the more well known surveys are the Epworth Sleepiness Questionnaire and the Berlin Questionnaire.

Questions on these tests might include gauging the chances that you'll doze off (not feel tired) in situations such as:

- Watching television

- Sitting and reading

- Sitting inactive in a public place such as a meeting

- As a passenger in a car for longer than one continuous hour

- Sitting and talking to someone

- Sitting quietly after a lunch without alcohol

- In a car while stopped for traffic

Other evaluative methods include assessing sleep habits as well as taking physical factors into account, as is the case with the STOP-BANG Questionnaire, with the name of the test standing for "snoring, tired, observed pressure, body mass index, age, neck circumference, and gender."

Additional evaluation methods could include a cephalometric analysis, to identify any growth abnormalities that may be affecting breathing, a Cone Beam CT Analysis to measure minimum airway volume, an intraoral evaluation to check for any potential visible obstructions, or a take home sleep monitor to measure key parameters like blood oxygen saturation, apnea and hypopnea episodes, and disturbed breathing patterns.

If one or more of these screenings do confirm the risk of OSA, the next step is a supervised sleep study monitored by a polysomnograph (PSG).

While a PSG will measure dozens of factors while the patient is sleeping, one of the most important factors it will be measuring is the person's apnea-hypopnea index, or AHI. This measurement determines exactly how many apneas, or pauses in breathing, the patient experiences in an hour, as well as moments of shallow breathing called hypopneas. Additionally, the study will count the number of respiratory effort-related arousals that patient experiences within an hour's time.

These measurements, along with accounts of the patient's heart rate, airflow, air pressure in the esophagus, oxygen saturation, snoring, eye movement, and even carbon dioxide levels of the skin, are taken into account before presenting the patient with a diagnosis.

OSA is a significant risk factor for:

- cardiovascular disease

- angina

- high blood pressure

- high cholesterol

- stroke

- type 2 diabetes

- asthma

- reflux

- depression

- memory loss

- irritability

- drowsiness while driving

- erectile dysfunction

Treating Obstructive Sleep Apnea

This is where dentists can play a significant role in treating or even curing OSA. If the condition is caused by a restricted airway, then the patient may benefit from oral appliance therapy.

There are several options for oral appliances that help with sleep apnea, and all of them are designed to hold the lower jaw forward, which creates a larger space between the base of the tongue and the back of the throat. If a patient is experiencing constriction at night, this adjustment should help keep that area more clear.

However, since oral appliances generally rely on the teeth to do their job, they're not recommended for people with periodontal disease or TMJ issues, as the appliance may exacerbate the condition. There are also potential side effects of long term usage, including:

- dry mouth

- excessive salivation

- tooth discomfort

- gingival irritation

- jaw muscle tenderness

- TMJ discomfort

- changes in bite due to teeth shifting from the pressure placed on them by the appliance. *

*This last side effect can often be managed by wearing a tooth positioner—a device that resembles a large sports mouth guard—for twenty to thirty minutes per day to keep the patients' teeth in their original position.

If oral appliances aren't an option, then the most common treatment for the condition is a continuous positive airway pressure device, or CPAP, which blows compressed air into the patient's nose and/or mouth while sleeping. While the CPAP is considered the "gold standard" for OSA treatment, it's also the least tolerated, as the mask can be uncomfortable to wear, and the pressure on the airway can irritate the nasal and upper airway tissues. Other options for treating sleep apnea, apart from lifestyle and behavior modification (losing weight, avoiding sleeping on the back, avoiding alcohol and/ or sedatives before bed, etc), may include:

- **Upper airway electrical stimulation**: a device that can be implanted in the chest to deliver mild electrical impulses to the nerve that controls the tongue, stimulating it to move when the patient stops breathing.

- **Maxillomandibular (double-jaw) advancement surgery**: for patients with significantly narrow airways, surgically moving the upper and lower jaws forward can help to open up the airway and tighten the muscles and tendons in those airways, reducing the risk of airway collapse.

- **Tonsillectomy and Adenoidectomy**: patients presenting with sleep apnea during childhood are more likely to benefit from these procedures, and have been shown to be highly effective in treating pediatric OSA.

- **Tracheostomy**: this procedure creates a small opening in the trachea below an obstruction in the airway. This procedure is usually only done in extreme cases of OSA, when no other options are available.

- **Nasal procedures**: if sleep apnea is mainly due to restrictions in the nasal area, surgeries can be conducted to address the blockage.

- **Uvulopalatopharyngoplasty**: This is a big word for an interesting procedure, which involves removing a portion of the soft palate around the uvula (that fleshy tissue hanging down in the back of the mouth) in order to open up the airway. While this can help with snoring, however, it's typically not as effective as other surgeries and therapies for treating OSA.

Now is the best time for preventative dental care

It never hurts to remind yourself that your dental health down the road depends on how healthy you keep your teeth today. As you age, any problems you have today are going to get worse unless they're treated, and neglect today can result in new issues and problems tomorrow. Overall health can go downhill fast, and keeping your mouth young in old age requires diligence; brushing and flossing twice a day are more important than ever, and keeping regular dental appointments will ultimately cost you much less in the long run, as failing to see the dentist could mean bigger—and costlier—dental conditions down the road.

In addition, remember those conditions that have been linked in one way or another to overall mouth health—diabetes, heart disease, stroke and respiratory problems have all been tied to the risk of bacteria from gum infections slipping directly into the bloodstream and triggering inflammation in organs and tissues.

Want to make it into your golden years with as many of your own, real teeth as possible? Then today is the best day to start a proper dental care routine that will last you the rest of your life.

Chapter Twelve

AGES 60+

Cavities and lost teeth are a serious issue at this age, in part due to the long-term wear and tear on gums and teeth that has already taken place.

With an average bite of two hundred pounds of pressure per square inch, the human mouth is pretty powerful, but that power also has the ability to wear down on the outer layer of tooth enamel over time. And when you combine a lifetime of chewing and grinding along with exposure to damaging acidic foods and drinks, you run the risk of more cracks, breaks, cavities and overall damage due to that weakened enamel.[35]

Gum recession, too, is more common in older adults, with a little more than 70 percent of people over the age of fifty showing some

---

35   "The aging mouth – and how to keep it younger," Harvard Health Publishing, Harvard Medical School, last modified January 2010, https://www.health.harvard. edu/diseases-and-conditions/the-aging-mouth-and-how-to-keep-it-younger

degree of recession, and 90 percent with signs of recession over the age of eighty.[36] When this condition is left untreated, the exposed root is more susceptible to gum disease, which could eventually lead to the destruction of the gum tissue and even the bone around the teeth.

Although there's not much you can do to stop the natural wearing down of tooth enamel, keeping up with daily dental health habits such as brushing, flossing, and regular dental visits are as important as ever at this age.

Toothbrushing a Challenge? Go Electric!

Daily habits that we used to do without a thought can become more burdensome in our later years. Just brushing teeth, for instance, can be difficult if arthritis or other disabilities affecting motor skills are beginning to manifest. For those with limited dexterity, switching from a manual toothbrush to an electric one can make a big difference. Additionally, switching to fluoride toothpastes that aid in the remineralization of the teeth can help strengthen tooth enamel and fill in the weak areas that plaque tends to cling to.

Dry Mouth (xerostomia)

Because of the prevalence of medications being taken in this age range, for conditions ranging from diabetes to blood pressure to cancer treatment, dry mouth is a common occurrence. Not only does this usually result in bad breath, but the lack of the mouth's natural cleanser—saliva—means that cavities are starting to come back into

---

36   Claudia Hammond, "Is age the cause of receding gums?" BBC Future, last modified August 7, 2013, http://www.bbc.com/future/story/20130807-does-age-damage-your-gums

play, and habits to combat the condition, such as sucking on sugary cough drops or hard candies, aren't helping the situation.

Dry mouth can also be a problem for denture wearers, as the lack of saliva can make the dentures feel loose in the mouth, leading to discomfort. In these cases, a denture fixative and/or artificial saliva can help, as can drinking sips of water frequently throughout the day. Other options for combating dry mouth include:

- Chewing sugarless gum

- Sucking on sugarless candies

- Avoiding alcohol or caffeinated beverages

- Avoiding tobacco

Varnish for a Healthier Smile

Even though cavities may seem like something only kids have to worry about, the fact is that the rate of tooth decay for people ages sixty-five-plus is now exceeding the rate of cavities in schoolchildren.[37] Part of this is due to those two age-related conditions mentioned earlier: dry mouth and gum recession. As the lack of self-cleaning saliva becomes more prevalent and more of that soft root tissue becomes exposed, the risk of developing cavities increases, particularly along the gum line.

To get ahead of that risk, more dentists are beginning to recommend a fluoride varnish around the base, or neck, of the teeth. The varnish, which usually consists of anywhere between .1 percent and 5 percent sodium fluoride and a resin or synthetic base that helps it stick to the teeth, sets rapidly and can be applied quickly, reducing

---

37 "The aging mouth – and how to keep it younger," Harvard Health Publishing, Harvard Medical School, last modified January 2010, https://www.health.harvard.edu/diseases-and-conditions/the-aging-mouth-and-how-to-keep-it-younger

the time that the hygienist spends in the mouth and minimizing the risk of gagging or accidental swallowing of the product.

While the majority of studies into the effectiveness of fluoride varnishes in preventing cavities have been conducted on children, more researchers are beginning to look into its impact on older adults. For children, systematic reviews have proven how effective topical fluoride can be in preventing or slowing the progress of cavities. With older adults, recent reviews have also shown a reduction in root cavities, with fluoride varnish controlling root cavities better than brushing with a high fluoride toothpaste alone. The study concluded that fluoride varnishes on older adults, particularly those who have difficulty brushing, would benefit from varnish being applied to the base of the teeth three to four times a year.[38]

Dental Implants and Dentures

More and more, implants are becoming the norm over dentures when it comes to replacing missing teeth. There are multiple reasons why— the main one being that implants look and act like real teeth. This doesn't just mean being able to tear into a corn-on-the-cob anytime you want—it also applies to how the implant acts in the mouth.

With dentures, the offending teeth are removed from the mouth and nothing replaces them. Over time, the body reabsorbs the bone that the teeth were removed from since it's no longer supporting teeth, leading to the degradation and thinning of the jaw. Implants, however, are made with a material that bonds with the bone, acting like real teeth so that the body isn't stimulated to begin reabsorption.

---

38   Nicola Innes and Dafydd Evans, "Caries prevention for older people in residential care homes," *Evidence-Based Dentistry* 10, no. 3 (2009): 83–87, https://doi. org/10.1038/sj.ebd.6400672

Other benefits include comfort—implants act like real teeth instead of shifting in the mouth or requiring fixatives, as dentures do—and longevity. The typical implant has a failure rate of less than 5 percent and lasts an average of twenty-five years, with some said to last a lifetime. Meanwhile, the lifecycle of dentures is usually anywhere from seven to fifteen years.[39]

Implants are also a healthier option for the surrounding teeth, as well. When a bridge is placed, for instance, the two teeth adjacent to the area need to ground down so that they can hold the bridge structure. Consequently, these newly worn teeth are more vulnerable to decay and damage.

How are Implants Implanted?

The implant procedure typically involves placing a titanium screw in just the right place in the jawbone, followed by the attachment of the prosthetic tooth. In some cases, patients may opt for a combination of implant and denture, in which a series of titanium screws are implanted in the jaw, with the external end shaped so that a partial or full denture can be snapped onto it.

Implants don't work for all patients, however. If you smoke, have diabetes, or have substantial bone loss already, implants may not be the best option.

---

39   Lesley Alderman, "For Most, Implants Beat Dentures, but at a Price," Health, The New York Times, last modified July 30, 2010, http://www.nytimes.com/2010/07/31/health/31patient.html

What to Know Before Whitening Older Teeth

As the outer layer of enamel thins, the dentin underneath becomes more visible, making teeth appear less white. Coffee, red wine, tea, and tobacco can also stain teeth, leading them to potentially look older than they are.

While over-the-counter whitening products and whitening toothpastes can help lighten teeth by a few shades, the effects are often much less dramatic in older teeth. However, before going through with a full-on dental whitening, keep in mind that professional whitening procedures may leave teeth feeling more sensitive and some stains may be more challenging to remove than others, requiring several rounds of bleaching before they can be removed.

Are Teeth Affected by Osteoporosis?

Osteoporosis, a medical condition that decreases the density of bones and makes them more likely to fracture, can also affect the bone density in the mouth. According to a study by the National Institute of Health, women with osteoporosis were three times more likely to have a loose tooth than women without the condition.[40]

Watching Out for Signs of Oral Cancer

As is the case with most cancers, the risk of oral cancer increases with age and the use of tobacco products. With each year that someone smokes or chews tobacco, the risk of developing oral cancer increases.

When oral cancer does develop, it's most likely to develop on the lower lip first, followed by the upper lip and then the tongue. Initial

---

40 "Oral Health and Bone Disease," NIH Osteoporosis and Related Bone Diseases National Resource Center, https://www.bones.nih.gov/health-info/bone/bone-health/oral-health/oral-health-and-bone-disease

signs and symptoms of the disease are easy to miss, but if you notice a white or red patch on your lip, tongue, or bottom of your mouth that lasts longer than two weeks, let your dentist know about it. While it may be the early signs of oral cancer, there's also the chance that it could be a sore caused by herpes or yeast infection, which, while painful, can also be treated.

Dental Care and Dementia

Older adults suffering from forms of dementia such as Alzheimer's disease should be allowed to conduct their own dental care for as long as they can, with reminders from family and caregivers, and supervision if needed. Establishing a daily care routine in the early stages of dementia is particularly important as assistance in brushing teeth may be needed later on.

Since it can often be challenging to communicate with someone who has dementia, it may be hard to tell if that person is suffering from mouth pain or discomfort. If you're a caregiver or family member of someone with dementia, it can help to keep an eye out for the following signs of potential dental problems:

- Refusing to eat hot or cold foods, or any food

- Frequent pulling at the face and mouth

- Increased moaning, shouting, or restlessness

- Refusal to take part in daily activities

- Aggressive behavior

- Disturbed sleep

- Not wearing dentures[41]

Dental Treatment for those Suffering from Dementia

According to the Alzheimer's Society, dental treatment for those suffering from dementia should be considered with all of the stages of dementia in mind. During the early stages, for instance, dentists should recommend and conduct treatment with the understanding that the patient will not be able to care for his or her own teeth at some point. Therefore, preventative treatments for conditions such as gum disease are very important. As the disease progresses, patients may need sedation or general anesthesia for dental visits, and their ability to co-operate during these visits should be assessed beforehand. In the late stages of dementia, the challenges of thinking clearly along with physical frailty and often additional complex medical conditions can make dental visits challenging, and care should mainly focus on maintaining the patient's comfort, preventing dental disease, and providing emergency treatment.[42]

When considering dental treatment for dementia patients, the following factors should be kept in mind:

- What dental problems are being experienced

- Whether the patient is able to give informed consent

- The patient's level of independence, thinking abilities, physical impairments, co-operation and mental state.

---

41   "Dental Care," Alzheimer's Society, https://www.alzheimers.org.uk/info/20029/daily_living/9/dental_care/3

42   Ibid.

Once these conditions are assessed, the dentist can provide input on the best treatment options for the patient, and how regularly he or she should see the dentist.

As with every stage of life, keeping teeth in their best condition requires regular maintenance and common sense practices. With this in mind, a little effort now can make a big difference in the teeth you get to keep—and their overall health—down the road.

For more information, or if you'd like to book an appointment, please call us at (613) 836-9084, contact us by email at Info@VillanovaDental.com, or visit our website at www.VillanovaDental.com.

Printed in the USA
CPSIA information can be obtained
at www.ICGtesting.com
JSHW012040140824
68134JS00033B/3164